EMOTIONAL AIKIDO: THE 2A + 2B + 2C + 2D SYSTEM

From Inner Conflict to Inner Harmony

Editing and Proofreading: Randy Saborit Mora
Interior Design, Cover Design and Layout: Otane González Martínez

La Fe Medical Clinic provides medical services and publishes educational and self-help books in the fields of mental health and general medicine, with a human-centered and accessible approach. For more information on how to obtain copies or access additional resources related to emotional health or medical services, please visit our websites:

La Fe Medical Clinic
3030 East 4th Street
Los Angeles, CA 90063

www.emotionalaikidomethod.com
www.lafeclinic.com
www.telegalenos.com

The book ***Emotional aikido: the 2A + 2B + 2C + 2D System*** *is part of the* ***Tools of Modern Psychiatry*** *collection. Through the 2A + 2B + 2C + 2D framework, readers learn to work with emotion —rather than against it— transforming internal conflict into adaptation, control and change.*

Emotional Aikido: the 2A + 2B + 2C + 2D System
Writeen by the Dr. Alexis Gómez González
ISBN: 978-1-968561-12-3

EMOTIONAL AIKIDO: THE 2A + 2B + 2C + 2D SYSTEM

Alexis Gómez González

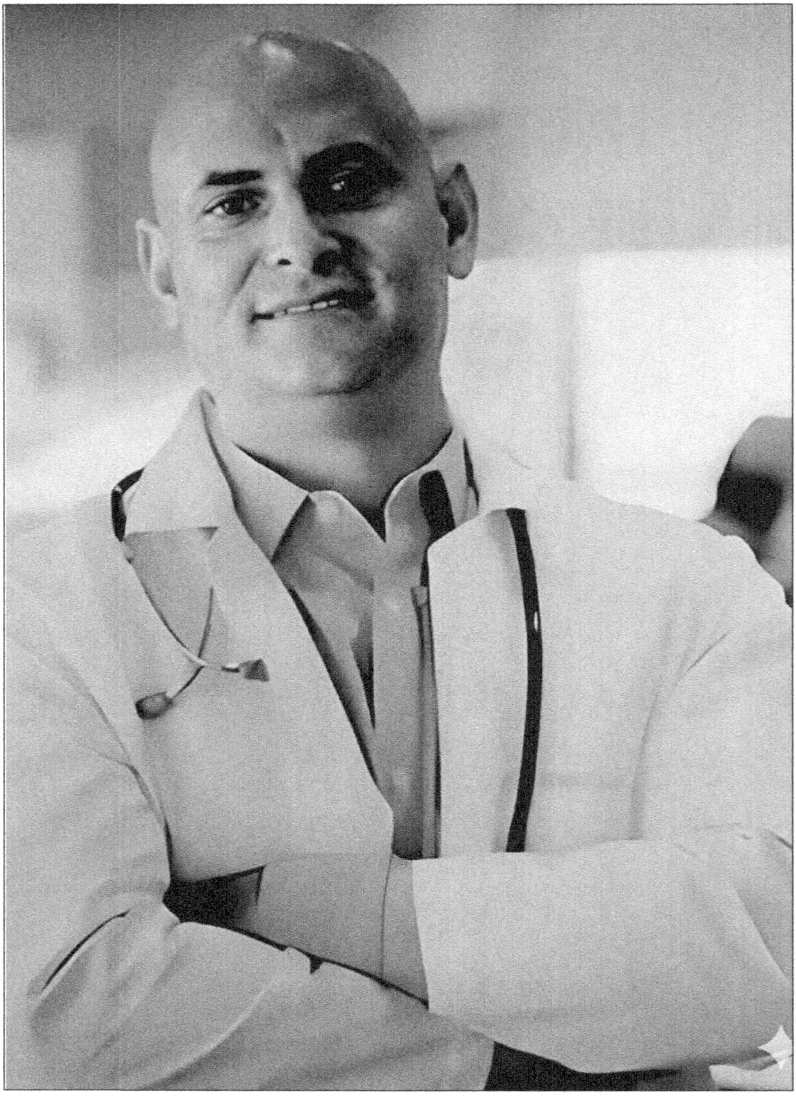

Author's presentation

My name is Alexis Gómez González. I am a physician who graduated from the School of Medical Sciences of Havana and from the University of Long Beach, California, with a specialty and a master's degree in family medicine and psychiatry. With more than 26 years of clinical, community, and teaching experience in Cuba, Mexico, and the United States, I have worked in the fields of family medicine and psychiatry in diverse communities across these countries, dedicating my career to humanizing medicine and bringing it closer to those who need it most.

I have built my professional life around the comprehensive and compassionate care of individuals with mental health disorders, with particular emphasis on anxiety, depression, insomnia, addictions, and neurodevelopmental disorders. Trained in both medicine and psychiatry, I have combined clinical knowledge with a strong passion for teaching and accessible dissemination.

I have created innovative graphic materials and have helped patients, families, and health professionals understand the complexity of the human mind in a clear and empathetic way. I have also worked on developing an approach that integrates science, compassion, and visual language as therapeutic and educational tools.

I currently direct one clinic in Los Angeles and another in Mexico City, both focused on the humanistic and effective treatment of psychiatric conditions, especially in vulnerable populations. I also participate in medical training projects, the creation of illustrated books, and community-based care initiatives.

Acknowledgements

This book would not have been possible without the support and contributions of many people. We are deeply grateful to the mental health professionals, researchers, and experts who shared their knowledge and experience to enrich the content of this work.

We also thank our editor and collaborators, whose effort and dedication made the publication of this book possible. Their support was fundamental at every stage of the process.

Finally, we thank all readers who seek to understand and cultivate their emotional intelligence. Your commitment to learning and growth is inspiring and essential to advancing projects and books like this one.

Index

Prologue

The Art of Winning without Fighting: the Emotional Revolution of the 21st Century

For centuries, humanity has learned how to fight. To fight nature. To fight others. To fight time. And perhaps the most silent and exhausting battle of all: to fight itself.

We fight fear when it appears without permission. We fight anger when it overflows the body. We fight sadness when it does not fit what we believe we *should* feel. We fight anxiety, emotional pain, and everything that seems beyond our control.

Without realizing it, this constant inner battle has become one of the greatest sources of psychological suffering in our time.

This book is born from a simple yet profound question: What if the problem is not the emotion itself... but the way we fight against it? Emotional Aikido proposes a radical shift in perspective.

It is not about repressing, dominating, or eliminating what we feel. It is about learning to move *with* emotion, just as in traditional Aikido: using the energy that arrives, redirecting it with awareness, and transforming impact into balance.

Winning without fighting does not mean surrender. It means letting go of unnecessary battles. It means using the intelligence of the body, the mind, and human connection to transform inner conflict into functional harmony. This is the emotional revolution of the 21st century.

For decades, emotional intelligence has been presented mainly as a cognitive skill: recognizing emotions, naming them, managing them. It has been a valuable contribution —but an incomplete one. In real life and in clinical practice, many people know perfectly well what they feel... and yet they still react, become overwhelmed, shut down, or repeat the same emotional patterns. Why? Because emotion does not live only in the mind.

It lives in the nervous system, in breathing, in posture, in the body's automatic reflexes. It lives in ancient neural circuits designed for survival, not for rational reflection. Emotional Aikido emerges from the integration of three great traditions of knowledge that rarely engage in deep dialogue with one another:

Modern neuroscience, which shows us how emotions are activated in the brain and body, how the amygdala responds before conscious thought, and how the vagus nerve, breathing, and posture regulate our internal state.

Contemporary psychotherapy, which has demonstrated that intellectual insight alone is not enough; emotional regulation must be experienced, trained, and transformed into sustainable internal habits.

And Eastern philosophy —particularly Aikido— which has long taught a truth often forgotten in the West: force is not met with force; energy is not blocked, it is redirected. From this integration arises the 2A + 2B + 2C + 2D system: eight emotional gates that transform the way we relate to what we feel and to those around us:

Anticipate.
Analyze.
Be welcome.
Benevolence.
Control.
Change.
Defeat.
Dissolve.

These are not abstract ideas. They are internal movements. They are bodily, emotional, and cognitive choices that can be trained, practiced, and strengthened over time. Unlike many self-help approaches, Emotional Aikido does not promise to eliminate uncomfortable emotions or to achieve a permanent state of calm. Life does not work that way. Emotions will continue to appear — sometimes intensely, sometimes without warning.

The difference lies in what we do when they appear. Emotional Aikido does not seek "perfectly balanced" people. It seeks *present* people. People who can feel without losing themselves.

Who can experience anger without destroying. Who can set boundaries without guilt.

Who can close conflicts without carrying resentment for years. At the heart of this method are four pillars that support the entire system:

Awareness, understood not only as mental insight, but as bodily perception —the ability to notice early signals, subtle shifts, and micro-changes that announce a reaction before it explodes.

Compassion, not as weakness, but as an advanced form of strength. Compassion toward oneself and toward others, recognizing that each person acts from their own level of regulation and their own wounds.

Control, not as emotional repression, but as conscious direction of inner energy. To control is to pause, breathe, adjust posture, and return to center before responding.

And Change, as the capacity for emotional flexibility —the ability to transform thoughts, habits, and automatic interpretations that keep us trapped in the same conflicts over and over again.

This book is not written only for therapists or mental health professionals. It is written for anyone who has ever felt overwhelmed by their emotions. For those who love, work, raise children, lead, make mistakes, and try again. For those who want to stop reacting and begin responding.

Throughout these pages you will find science, yes —but also humanity. You will find clear explanations, but above all, you will find practices designed for real life: at work, in relationships, in families, in moments of crisis, and in everyday silence.

Emotional Aikido is not a technique for "winning arguments". It is a path to inner coherence. It is not about controlling others. It is about reclaiming your own center.

If this book helps you, in your next difficult moment, to pause for a single second instead of reacting impulsively —to breathe and choose a more conscious movement— then it has already fulfilled its purpose.

Because the true art of winning without fighting is not about mastering the world, but about learning to inhabit it with greater clarity, dignity, and inner peace.

Dr. Alexis Gómez González

PART I.
The Art of Inner Energy

CHAPTER 1.
Emotional Aikido: the New Art of Mastering Inner Energy

1.1 The Silent Revolution

The twenty-first century has changed the way we live, feel, and think. We no longer fight for food or territory, but for something far more subtle: emotional stability, meaning, and genuine connection.

The fiercest battle is no longer fought in the streets or in temples —it is fought within every human mind. We live in an age of overstimulation: screens that demand attention, opinions that divide, rhythms that leave no space to breathe.

The body tightens, the mind reacts, and the soul —that quiet part still longing for coherence— asks how to remain at peace without withdrawing from the world. The answer is neither resistance nor escape. The answer is **Emotional Aikido**.

1.2 The Birth of a New Intelligence

Since Daniel Goleman introduced *Emotional Intelligence*, we've known that success and fulfillment depend more on how we understand and manage emotions than on pure intellect. But understanding is not the same as transformation. We can know we are angry and still lose control. We can recognize anxiety and still let it paralyze us. We can preach calm and still live enslaved by reactivity.

Emotional intelligence was the first step. **Emotional Aikido** is the next. It is embodied, dynamic, and practical emotional intelligence —a discipline that doesn't merely analyze emotion but moves, redirects, and dissolves it with elegance and purpose.

1.3 From the Dojo to the Heart

Aikido, created by Morihei Ueshiba, is a martial art without attack —a movement of peace in the midst of chaos. The aikidoka doesn't seek to defeat the opponent but to transform himself while redirecting conflict toward harmony. Violence is dissolved through motion. The enemy becomes the teacher.

In **Emotional Aikido**, the dojo is internal. Each emotion is a symbolic opponent that, once recognized, reveals its hidden message. There are no punches, only lessons. No resistance, only flow. No enemies, only energy waiting to be understood. The body, mind, and emotion merge into a single choreography—and in that conscious dance, chaos turns to balance.

1.4 The Eight Gates of Balance: The 2A + 2B + 2C + 2D System

Every emotion is energy in motion. When it flows, it propels us forward. When it stagnates, it becomes suffering. The **2A + 2B + 2C + 2D** system proposes eight internal movements to redirect that energy toward harmony—the emotional map of the inner aikidoka:

- **Anticipate:** perceive the signs before the impulse takes over.
- **Analyze:** understand the origin, intention, and meaning of the emotion.
- **Be welcome:** open the door to what you feel without denial or resistance.

- **Benevolence:** respond with empathy, compassion, and inner strength.
- **Control:** stabilize the body, breath, and mind.
- **Change:** reprogram thought and behavior consciously.
- **Defeat:** break toxic cycles without harming anyone.
- **Dissolve:** release the emotional charge and return to equilibrium.

These eight gates form a sequence of emotional transformation—a flow from feeling to understanding, from containment to liberation. They are the art of turning every inner impact into wisdom.

1.5 Science and Spirituality in One Gesture

Emotional Aikido unites two languages that rarely meet: neuroscience and spirituality.

Each internal movement has a precise physiological correlate:

- **Anticipate:** activates the insular cortex, the brain's emotional radar.
- **Analyze:** engages the hippocampus and prefrontal cortex, where meaning is created.
- **Be welcome:** stimulates oxytocin —the hormone of openness and connection.
- **Benevolence:** modulates the ventromedial prefrontal cortex, seat of empathy and moral calm.
- **Control:** regulates the vagus nerve, slowing the heart and steadying the body.
- **Change:** strengthens the dorsolateral cortex, the center of cognitive reframing.
- **Defeat:** activates the anterior cingulate cortex, which interrupts reactive patterns.
- **Dissolve:** synchronizes the default mode network, restoring serenity.

Yet beyond biology lies purpose.Emotional Aikido teaches that to feel is not a failure but an opportunity for evolution.

Fear protects.
Anger defends.
Sadness purifies.
Guilt teaches.
Joy integrates.
Serenity reveals.
Each emotion is a message, not a threat.

1.6 The New Warrior

The old warrior mastered the outer world; the new one masters the inner. His sword is awareness. His armor is calm. His victory is peace. Emotional Aikido doesn't aim to eliminate conflict but to transform it into growth.

It doesn't erase anger —it converts it into clarity. It doesn't suppress fear —it channels it into prudence. It doesn't flee from pain —it turns it into wisdom. To practice Emotional Aikido is to walk toward a new humanity —more present, more conscious, more kind.

It is the invisible training of leaders, healers, parents, and awake souls who understand that true power is not imposed but radiated.

1.7 The Promise

This book doesn't promise a life without emotion. It promises a life where emotion becomes a teacher, not a tyrant. Where every impulse turns into a movement of awareness. Where mind and heart stop fighting and begin to dance together.

Emotional Aikido is not a technique —it is a path. A journey toward inner harmony that begins with a single gesture: **welcoming what you feel**. And in that welcome, transformation begins.

CHAPTER 2.
The Neurophysiology of Emotional Flow

2.1 The Architecture of Emotion

Emotions are not random storms; they are the most refined survival mechanism the human brain has ever produced. Each feeling, from fear to joy, is a precise biochemical signal—a bridge between body and mind, past and present, perception and action.

Three great systems work together every time you feel:

1- The Limbic System, the emotional brain, detects relevance, danger, or opportunity. The amygdala sounds the alarm, the hippocampus recalls similar experiences, and the hypothalamus prepares the body for reaction.

2- The Autonomic Nervous System translates that alarm into physiological reality —faster heartbeat, shallow breathing, changes in blood flow.

3- The Prefrontal Cortex, seat of reasoning and planning, interprets and regulates. It decides whether that emotion becomes chaos or clarity.

The ancient and the modern coexist within us: the reptilian impulse to survive and the human capacity to observe ourselves in real time. Emotional Aikido is the art of reconciling both—of allowing instinct to move and consciousness to guide.

2.2 The 90-Second Window

When neuroscientist Jill Bolte Taylor observed her own brain under the effects of a stroke, she discovered a remarkable truth: the chemical surge of an emotion—adrenaline, cortisol, and neurotransmitter changes— lasts about **90 seconds**.

After that, the emotion's biological wave naturally subsides. What prolongs suffering is not chemistry —it's repetition. It's the mind replaying the story, the thought reactivating the same neural circuit again and again.

In Emotional Aikido, those 90 seconds are sacred. They are your inner dojo, your window of transformation. In that short span, you can breathe, ground, and redirect. You can let the emotion pass through you without identifying with it. It's the space between reaction and response—the birthplace of freedom.

2.3 The Body as an Emotional Mirror

Every emotion is written on the body.

- **Anger** tightens the jaw and fists, mobilizing muscles for defense.
- **Fear** contracts the diaphragm, preparing for flight or freeze.
- **Sadness** lowers the shoulders and slows the breath, inviting introspection.
- **Joy** opens the chest and lifts the eyes, signaling safety.

The body doesn't lie; it reveals what the mind hides. Learning to read it is learning to listen to the language of the subconscious.

Aikido calls this unity **Shin-Tai-Ichi** —the oneness of mind and body. Modern science calls it **interoception**— the capacity to perceive internal sensations and use them as data.

To "feel" your emotion is not weakness; it's neurobiological mastery. The earlier you detect its physical trace, the earlier you can apply the two A's: **Anticipate** and **Analyze**.

2.4 The Emotional Flow: from Energy to Awareness

The emotional process is a cycle of energy that moves through predictable stages. Each stage aligns with one step of the **2A + 2B + 2C +2D** system and with specific neural pathways:

Stage	Brain / Body System	Function
Anticipate	Insular cortex + prefrontal awareness	Early detection of emotional shifts
Analyze	Prefrontal cortex + hippocampus	Cognitive labeling and meaning-making
Be welcome	Oxytocin and mirror neuron systems	Emotional acceptance and social safety
Benevolence	Ventromedial prefrontal cortex	Compassion and moral regulation
Control	Vagus nerve and parasympathetic activation	Autonomic balance and grounding
Change	Dorsolateral prefrontal cortex	Cognitive reappraisal and habit shift
Defeat	Anterior cingulate cortex	Conflict monitoring and interruption of reactivity
Dissolve	Default mode network	Integration and emotional closure

This is not abstract philosophy—it is neuroscience in motion. Every time you apply one of these steps, your brain reorganizes.

You train new pathways, strengthen new habits, and teach your nervous system that peace is a choice, not an accident.

2.5 The Vagus Nerve: the Hidden Conductor

If there were a single instrument orchestrating emotional balance, it would be the **vagus nerve**. Extending from the brainstem to the heart, lungs, and intestines, it carries the signals of calm, safety, and presence.

When activated through slow breathing, mindful posture, or compassionate thought, the vagus nerve lowers heart rate, increases oxygen flow, and restores clarity to the mind. It is the biological foundation of **Control** and **Dissolve** —the bridge between the nervous system and serenity.

A calm vagus is not the absence of emotion —it is the capacity to feel deeply without being drowned.

2.6 Emotional Resonance and Synchrony

Human beings are resonant creatures. Our nervous systems synchronize with others through subtle signals: tone of voice, eye contact, rhythm of breathing. This is why one person's calm can pacify a room, and one person's rage can ignite it. **Emotional Aikido** uses this phenomenon consciously.

By cultivating internal coherence —through breath, posture, and benevolence— you radiate physiological stability. In teams, families, or therapy, this coherence becomes contagious: what begins as self-regulation becomes collective harmony.

2.7 The Circle of Transformation

Emotion begins in the body, moves through awareness, and returns as meaning. The loop completes when the feeling is integrated, not suppressed. The eight disciplines of Emotional Aikido correspond exactly to this journey: from impulse to insight, from instinct to wisdom. To master emotion is not to silence it —it is to let it complete its cycle. Like an Aikido movement, emotion has its natural arc: it rises, spirals, and returns to center.

2.8 From Science to Practice

Each breath, each pause, each deliberate thought rewires your brain. Neuroplasticity doesn't happen only in therapy rooms —it happens in every moment you choose awareness over reaction.

Emotional Aikido is therefore:

- **Philosophy:** non-resistance and compassion.
- **Science:** interoception, regulation, and neural integration.
- **Practice:** repetition, embodiment, and courage.

Every time you breathe consciously instead of exploding, every time you welcome emotion instead of denying it, you are performing an act of neurobiological mastery. You are proving that peace is not passivity —it is precision.

And so the dojo becomes invisible: your breath, your thoughts, your words. Every interaction becomes training. Every emotion becomes a chance to evolve.

CHAPTER 3.
Aikido of Grief: the Art of Falling without Breaking

3.1 Introduction

Every true loss produces a rupture. It is not only the loss of a person, a role, or a life stage; it is the loss of **a version of oneself**. Grief is the process through which the mind, the body, and identity attempt to reorganize after that break.

From the perspective of medical aikido, grief is not a disease that must be corrected nor a weakness that must be overcome quickly. It is **an inevitable movement**. And like all movement, it can be carried out clumsily—shattering internal structures—or with technique, awareness, and compassion.

Aikido teaches something essential: not every strike can be avoided, not every fall can be prevented. However, through aikido one can learn to fall without destroying oneself. This chapter integrates the model of the stages of grief described by **Elisabeth Kübler-Ross** with the logic of medical aikido and its **2A + 2B + 2C + 2D** formula, transforming grief into a process that is **accompanied, intelligible, and clinically safe**.

3.2 Grief Is not a Staircase, It Is a Wave

One of the most common mistakes —both clinical and personal— is to think that grief unfolds in orderly steps. In reality, grief resembles the sea: there are large waves, small waves, retreats, moments of apparent calm, and unexpected surges.

Aikido does not force the body to move in a straight line. It adapts to the flow. That is why it is an ideal framework for grief: it **respects emotional dynamics without imposing violence**.

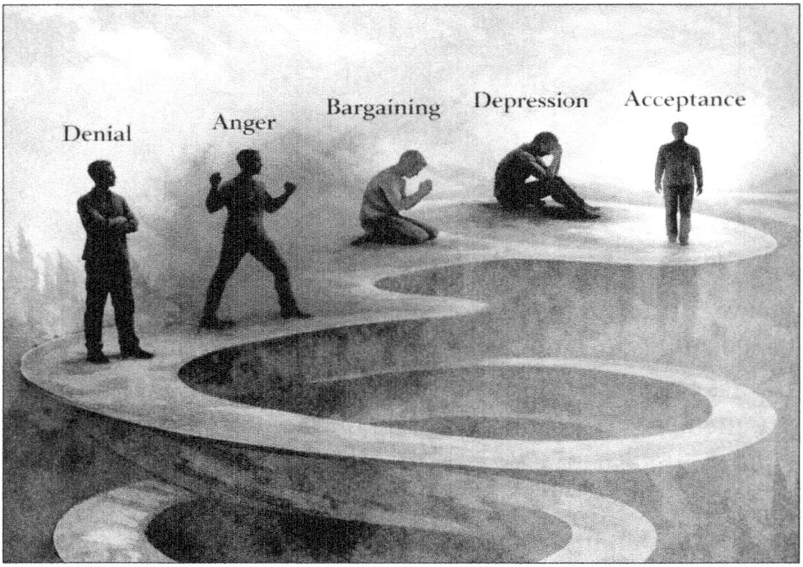

Figure 1. The stages of grief are not traveled in a straight line. Denial, anger, bargaining, depression, and acceptance emerge as successive —sometimes simultaneous— movements within the process of emotional integration. The aikido of grief proposes moving through them without violent resistance, learning how to fall without destroying oneself.

3.3 The Medical Aikido Formula Applied to Grief

2A: Anticipate and Analyze

Understanding which emotion will appear and why.

2B: Be Welcome and Benevolence

Allowing the experience without judgment or demand.

2C: Control and Change

Regaining the center and redirecting energy.

2D: Knock Down and Dissolve

Allowing the fall and dissolving inner conflict.

Each stage of grief activates one or more of these principles:

1. Denial

Anticipate the fall, welcome it

Denial is often misinterpreted as immaturity or emotional coldness. In reality, it is a neuro-emotional protective mechanism. The mind doses reality when the impact is too great. From medical aikido: denial is not attacked, confronted, or ridiculed. Its appearance is anticipated and it is welcomed.

Example:

A woman loses her mother after a long illness. During the funeral she organizes everything with surgical precision; she smiles and comforts others. Days later she says, "I haven't cried at all, I'm fine".

The mistake would be to push her: "You still haven't accepted it." Aikido proposes something else: holding the space until the body is ready. Weeks later, she will cry —and she will do so without collapsing. Clinically, well-accompanied denial prevents later breakdowns.

2. Anger

Analyze the strike, use the energy

Anger is the moment when pain becomes directional. It is no longer shock; it is force. Many people are frightened when they pass through this phase because they feel they are "becoming bad." In aikido, force is not the enemy; it is raw material.

Analyzing anger involves asking:

- Which value was violated?
- Which bond was torn away?
- What injustice is being perceived?

Example:

A man loses his job after 20 years. He is not sad; he is furious. He feels betrayed and humiliated. He insults the company, his bosses, and himself.

The therapeutic task is not to extinguish anger but to redirect it. Rage becomes a boundary; the boundary becomes clarity; clarity becomes decision. When anger is used well, it restores the axis.

3. Bargaining

Control the center, change direction

Here adult magical thinking appears: "If I had done…", "If I do X, maybe Y won't be lost entirely". This is not stupidity; it is the mind trying to regain control. From medical aikido:

- The center is controlled without rigidity.
- Direction is changed without humiliating hope.

Example:

A father loses his child in an accident. He mentally repeats every past decision. He believes that if he had changed a single thing, everything would have been different. Aikido does not say, "That's irrational". It helps him release omnipotence without destroying love. When the illusion of absolute control dissolves, something healthier remains: responsibility without toxic guilt.

4. Depression

Learning to fall without breaking

Grief-related depression is not a mistake. It is the real weight of loss once active defenses are gone. The problem is not falling; the problem is falling badly. In aikido, falling is trained because falling is inevitable.

Example:

A retired woman—healthy and active—enters a deep sadness after losing her work role. She did not lose a person; she lost identity. She feels useless and invisible. She does not need forced motivation. She needs permission to fall without shame.

Here, the aikido of grief is based on:

- radical benevolence,
- minimal goals,
- constant presence.

One does not push upward. One prevents breaking further downward.

5. Acceptance

Dissolve the struggle, integrate the wound

Acceptance is not forgetting. It is not being at peace all the time. It is **stopping the fight** with reality. In aikido, when conflict dissolves, energy returns to the center.

Example:

A patient with a chronic illness understands that life will not return to what it was before. He is not happy about it, but he stops resisting. He begins to reorganize his identity. The loss ceases to be an open wound and becomes integrated memory.

2.4 Can Grief Be Traversed Faster?

The aikido of grief does not promise shortcuts. It promises **less damage**. For example, when one does not fight each emotion:

- There is less guilt.
- Less stagnation.
- Fewer complicated grief processes.

Grief is not artificially shortened, but it flows without **becoming entrenched**. Grief is not defeated. It is not overcome like an enemy. It is honored. It is traversed. It is integrated. The aikido of grief reminds us of something essential: **not everything that falls is lost**. Some things, when they fall well, are transformed.

When pain is no longer fought and is integrated with awareness, the wound ceases to be a rupture and becomes a source of growth. The aikido of grief does not teach how to avoid falling, but how to rise without destroying oneself. Not everything that breaks is lost. Some cracks let the light in.

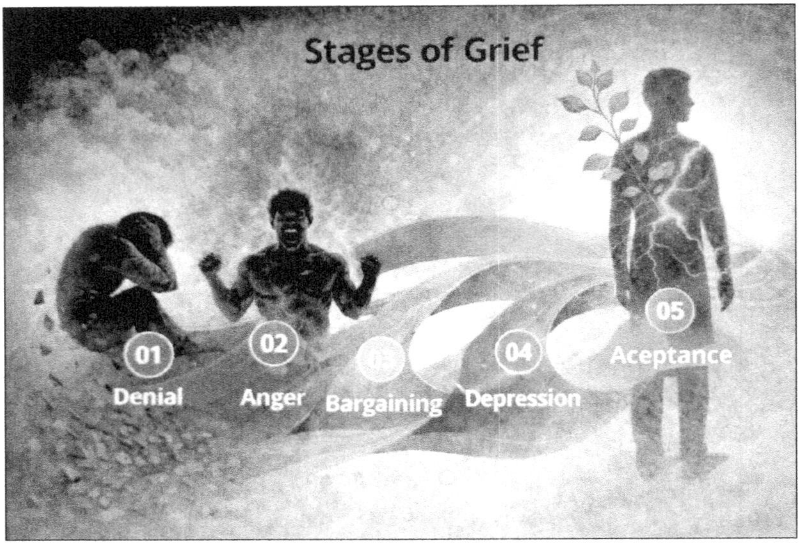

Figure 2. With medical aikido, grief does not disappear —it transforms.

PART II.
The Eight Disciplines of Emotional Aikido (2A + 2B + 2C + 2D)

CHAPTER 4.
Anticipate: the Radar of Emotional Awareness

4.1 Seeing Before Feeling

To anticipate is not to predict the future; it is to perceive the first echoes of the present. Most emotional conflicts don't erupt suddenly—they build quietly through micro-signals, gestures, and subtle tensions that the body detects long before the mind understands them.

The body always knows first. When you learn to anticipate, you stop being a victim of your emotions. Anger no longer surprises you because you recognize the warmth rising in your chest.

Anxiety no longer dominates you because you sense its vibration in your stomach. Sadness no longer drags you down because you detect its silence forming in your voice.

To anticipate is to become the observer of your own inner waves —to awaken sensory awareness before the reaction takes control. The emotional aikidoka never waits for the strike; he feels it coming, centers himself, and decides how to move.

4.2 The Neuroscience of Anticipation

The **insular cortex** is the organ of bodily intuition —the radar of the brain. It registers the subtlest changes in breathing, pulse, temperature, and muscle tension. When this region is active, we can notice emotions before they manifest.

Brain-imaging studies show that people with strong **interoceptive awareness** —the ability to feel what is happening inside their bodies— regulate anxiety, anger, and fear more effectively.
Their nervous systems recognize the first milliseconds of emotional change, and that interval becomes space for choice. In Emotional Aikido, anticipation is that microsecond between stimulus and reaction —the instant when consciousness can enter and redirect the flow.

4.3 The Body as an Antenna

Anticipation begins in the body, not in the analyzing mind but in the sensing organism.

The body constantly captures micro-signals:

- **Pulse:** a slight acceleration may indicate alertness or impatience.
- **Breathing:** if it shortens, the body is preparing to flee or defend.
- **Jaw:** if it tightens, something unsaid is demanding release.
- **Back:** if it slumps, fatigue or hidden sadness is present.
- **Skin:** goosebumps or flushing reveal a threat already detected by the nervous system.

Training the bodily radar is cultivating the inner dojo. Every muscle, every breath, every gesture becomes an instrument of emotional diagnosis.

4.4 The Map of Early Signals

The emotional aikidoka learns to build a *map of signals*—a record of the changes that precede his most common emotions.

Emotion	Bodily Signal	Initial Thought	Anticipatory Action
Anger	Warmth in chest, tight jaw	"This is unfair".	Deep breath + relax shoulders
Anxiety	Tight abdomen, short breath	"I can't handle this".	Three deep breaths + upright posture
Sadness	Lump in throat	"What's the point?"	Hand on chest + long exhale
Guilt	Downward gaze, neck tension	"It's my fault".	Recognize without judgment + compassionate phrase

This map is built through observation and writing. Each person has a unique bodily language. To anticipate means to become literate in your own biology.

4.5 Exercise 1: Conscious Body Scan (3 minutes)

1- Sit with your back straight and feet grounded.

2- Close your eyes and bring your attention inward.

3- Mentally scan from head to toes, noticing sensations—pressure, temperature, tension, tingling.

4- If something draws your attention, don't change it; simply **observe** and **name** it ("tension in neck," "warmth in chest").

5- Breathe gently into that area for three cycles.

This exercise strengthens the connection between the insula (emotional radar) and the prefrontal cortex (awareness). It is the first discipline of the emotional aikidoka.

4.6 Exercise 2: Anticipatory Breathing (90 seconds)

1- Before replying to a difficult message, entering a meeting, or facing conflict, **pause**.

2- Inhale through the nose for a count of **four**, hold for **two**, exhale through the mouth for **six**.

3- During the exhale, repeat mentally: "I feel, but I do not react".

4- Notice how the body's tone begins to change.

This technique activates the vagus nerve and expands the gap between stimulus and response. With practice, that gap becomes spacious enough to act with consciousness rather than impulse.

4.7 Exercise 3: Emotional Anticipation Journal (7 days)

For one week, record three daily moments:

- What you felt.
- What bodily signals appeared first.
- What you did to anticipate or regulate.
- What outcome you observed.

Example:

"Before feeling anger, I noticed heat in my neck and shallow breath. I anticipated the emotion, breathed deeply, and asked for a moment before answering. Result: I spoke without shouting".

Over time, this diary becomes a personalized emotional map —the intimate cartography of your nervous system.

4.8 The Power to Foresee without Controlling

To anticipate does not mean to avoid emotion; it means to meet it with lucidity. It's like reading the ocean before stepping into the waves. Knowing a wave is coming won't stop it —but it allows you to surf it.

The emotional aikidoka does not numb sensitivity; he refines it. The more sensitive he becomes, the faster he perceives change —and the freer his response. Anticipation is not fear of impact; it is love of balance.

4.9 The Mind as Observatory

When the body learns to anticipate, the mind learns to observe without interference. Pure observation dissolves identification with emotion. You stop saying "I am angry" and begin to notice "there is anger within me".

That subtle shift changes the entire brain dynamic: the amygdala quiets down, and the prefrontal cortex resumes command. This is the silent victory of the emotional aikidoka: not conquering emotion, but **conquering automatic reaction**.

4.10 The Lesson of the Chapter

Anticipation is the first gate of Emotional Aikido because it is the most preventive. It allows you to act before pain becomes injury, before reaction becomes habit, before impulse erases awareness.

True emotional intelligence doesn't begin when you control what you feel —it begins when you **notice** that you are about to feel. The emotional aikidoka does not live on guard; he lives attentive, serene, and present.

His body is a radar, his mind an observatory, his emotions pure information. And in that conscious anticipation, conflict loses its power.

CHAPTER 5.
Analyze: understanding the Hidden Message of Each Emotion

5.1 The Meaning Behind the Impact

Every emotion is a coded message. It doesn't arise to punish you —it arises to inform you. Emotions are the oldest language of the brain, biological signals that communicate needs, limits, memories, and lessons.

Anger doesn't appear to make you lose control —it appears to protect you when something feels unjust.

Fear doesn't arrive to paralyze you —it warns that something requires attention or caution. Sadness isn't weakness —it's a process of internal repair.

Guilt isn't punishment —it's a moral compass asking for correction. Even shame —so often misunderstood— tries to keep you connected to others, though it can easily distort its purpose.

To analyze is to **decode the message** your emotion is trying to send before it turns into suffering. Emotion only becomes toxic when it is not understood.

5.2 The Neuroscience of Emotional Interpretation

When an emotion is triggered, the brain sends information through three simultaneous levels:

1- **Physiological:** the body reacts (heartbeat, breathing, muscle tension).

2- **Cognitive:** the mind creates a story ("They're attacking me," "I'm not enough").

3- **Behavioral:** we act (yelling, fleeing, staying silent).

The key is to intervene in the second level —the interpretive thought. That's where the brain **assigns meaning** to what we feel. The **hippocampus** compares the new event to past experiences. The **amygdala** evaluates safety or threat. The **prefrontal cortex** decides what story to tell.

If the interpretation is realistic, the emotion flows and teaches. If it is distorted, it repeats and amplifies. Thus, analysis is not about rationalizing —it is about **giving conscious context** to emotion.

5.3 The Inner Observer

To analyze is to create a mental space where you can see what you feel without becoming it. It means saying to yourself, "I am feeling anger, but I am not anger. I am feeling fear, but I am not fear".
That distance —called **meta-awareness**— allows you to think clearly while the body feels intensely. The emotional aikidoka doesn't flee from the strike; he observes it in slow motion.
Analyzing is practicing that **inner movement** where awareness and emotion coexist without conflict.

5.4 Questions that Awaken Consciousness

To analyze an emotion, curiosity is required —not judgment. These questions act as keys to self-understanding:

1- What am I really feeling? (use a precise word).

2- When did this emotion begin?

3- What value or need feels threatened?

4- What thoughts accompany this sensation?

5- Where in my body is it located?

6- What might this emotion want to teach or protect right now?

Answering activates the prefrontal cortex—the brain area that transforms impulse into insight. Every time you name an emotion, you reduce its intensity: "Name it to tame it". Naming is the first act of mastery.

5.5 The Three-Cause Method

The emotional aikidoka uses a simple model to analyze emotions without drowning in them:

1. **Biological cause:** Am I tired, hungry, or in physical pain?
2. **Psychological cause:** What thought, memory, or expectation triggered it?
3. **Symbolic cause:** What does this emotion represent in my history or identity?

Example:

You feel anxiety before speaking in public.

- Biological: You slept poorly.
- Psychological: You fear making a mistake.
- Symbolic: As a child, you were humiliated for speaking up.

Analysis reveals that the current emotion is not just about the present moment —it is an echo of many past experiences. Recognizing that truth diminishes its power and lets you respond from adulthood rather than from the old wound.

5.6 Exercise 1: emotional Meaning Journal (5 minutes a day)

Each evening, choose one emotion you experienced that day and write:

- What you felt.
- What triggered it.

- What it was trying to teach or protect.
- What you learned from it.

Example:

"I felt anger when my message wasn't answered. Analyzing it, I realized it wasn't about the message but about feeling ignored. My true need was to feel valued".

Over time, this journal becomes a mirror of awareness—a living X-ray of the emotional self in motion.

5.7 Exercise 2: the Conversation with Emotion

Imagine your emotion can speak.
Close your eyes and say silently: "Hello, anger (or fear, sadness, guilt). I won't reject you. I want to understand why you've come".

Then listen to what arises —an image, a phrase, a memory, a sensation. This dialogue activates the brain's right hemisphere, responsible for empathy and imagination. It transforms the emotion from an enemy into a guide.

5.8 The Myth of Emotional Control

Control doesn't mean repression. Control without analysis becomes rigidity; analysis without control becomes chaos. Only by understanding the emotion can you direct it with elegance.

Cultures that glorify emotional suppression create tense bodies and exhausted minds. Those that worship raw expression breed impulsivity and drama. **Emotional Aikido** teaches the middle path: **understand in order to choose**.

5.9 The Therapeutic Order of Understanding

When you analyze an emotion clearly, something neurobiological happens:

The amygdala (center of fear) calms down, and the prefrontal cortex (reason and regulation) regains command.

The brain literally **switches modes** —from defense to learning. That is why emotional analysis is medicine. It doesn't just soothe; it reprograms. Each time you reflect instead of react, you forge a new neural bridge between emotion and wisdom.

5.10 The Lesson of the Chapter

Analyzing is the second gate of Emotional Aikido. If anticipating is perceiving movement, analyzing is **understanding its direction**.

Without analysis, emotion is noise. With analysis, it becomes music. Understanding your emotions is not intellectual weakness —it is spiritual maturity.

The emotional aikidoka knows that lucidity is his best defense: he does not react by impulse; he acts with purpose. And in doing so, he turns chaos into clarity, and emotion into knowledge.

CHAPTER 6.
Be welcome: transforming Emotion into an Ally

6.1 The Art of Emotional Welcome

Every emotion arrives like an unexpected guest —sometimes gentle, sometimes loud, sometimes terrifying. Most people respond by shutting the door.

They resist anger, avoid fear, and suppress sadness, believing that control means rejection. But what we resist, persists. What we welcome, transforms.

To be welcome is to open the door consciously and say: "I see you. You may enter, but you will not rule me".

That phrase defines the true power of Emotional Aikido: not domination, but inclusion.

Because every emotion —pleasant or painful— carries energy, memory, and a hidden intelligence that can be integrated into our growth.

When you welcome emotion, you dissolve the inner war between the part of you that feels and the part that fears feeling. In that reconciliation, you recover your unity.

6.2 From Resistance to Reception

The human brain naturally avoids discomfort.The amygdala interprets strong emotions as threats, and the body reacts with tension or escape.

But neuroscientific studies show that when we approach emotion with curiosity instead of resistance, the prefrontal cortex reactivates and the nervous system calms.

Acceptance is not passivity —it is regulation. It turns off the survival alarm and gives the body permission to process safely.

The moment you say inwardly, "It's okay to feel this", the chemistry changes: cortisol drops, oxytocin rises, and the body moves from defense to coherence. That simple inner phrase is both neurobiology and compassion in action.

6.3 The Meeting Point: Emotion and Consciousness

When a feeling appears —anger, shame, fear, grief— it's tempting to either analyze it immediately or push it away. Welcoming is the middle way: the pause that allows the emotion to reveal itself without judgment.

Imagine sitting in front of your feeling as if it were a visitor in need of attention. You don't interrogate or silence it; you listen. In that listening, the feeling begins to soften. This is the emotional equivalent of the Aikido movement called Irimi: entering the attack, not to fight it, but to blend with its trajectory until conflict dissolves.

6.4 The Physiology of Acceptance

When we welcome emotion, the body changes in measurable ways:

- The **ventromedial prefrontal cortex** reduces the amygdala's alarm.
- The **vagus nerve** activates, slowing the heart and deepening breath.
- The **oxytocin system** releases feelings of safety and trust.
- The **insula** increases awareness of inner sensations.

This is the neurophysiology of serenity: emotional acceptance as a biological act of healing. The ancient wisdom of "what you embrace, heals" now has scientific proof.

6.5 Exercise 1: the Inner Welcome (2 minutes)

1- Close your eyes. Inhale deeply through your nose and exhale slowly through your mouth.

2- Notice what emotion is present right now —without naming it "good" or "bad".

3- Place one hand on your chest and say inwardly: "You are welcome here. I will listen".

4- Breathe three times as if each breath made more space inside you.

5- Simply stay. No fixing, no judging, no analyzing.

This exercise retrains the nervous system to experience intensity without panic. It's emotional exposure therapy guided by compassion.

6.6 Exercise 2: Dialogue of Integration

After a conflict or a stressful day, take a notebook and write a conversation between you and the emotion that dominated the event.

Example:

You: "Anger, you came so fast today. What were you protecting?"

Anger: "Your boundaries. You felt unseen".

You: "Thank you. Next time, tell me earlier—I'll listen sooner".

This exercise reprograms the emotional memory. You move from suppression to dialogue, from reactivity to alliance.

6.7 The Psychology of Inclusion

In psychotherapy, emotions are treated as signals of unmet needs. Rejection of emotion equals rejection of need. Welcoming it restores the bridge between psyche and soma—between the feeling and the body that feels.

Many people fear that if they welcome sadness, it will consume them; that if they welcome anger, it will destroy them. But it is the resistance, not the emotion itself, that causes suffering. The unaccepted emotion becomes a ghost haunting the nervous system.

To welcome emotion is to **complete its biological cycle**. Once acknowledged, the brain stops sending the alarm signal.

6.8 The Compassion Reflex

In Emotional Aikido, welcoming is not just acceptance —it's benevolence in motion. When you welcome an emotion, you practice compassion toward yourself. You stop treating feelings as intruders and begin to see them as messengers of care.

This act activates the **social engagement system:** a network connecting the vagus nerve, facial muscles, and heart rhythm.

That's why a compassionate inner attitude literally changes your face, your tone, your presence. Others feel it. Emotional coherence is contagious.

6.9 The Inner Bow

In traditional Aikido, practitioners bow to one another before training —a gesture of respect, gratitude, and humility.

In Emotional Aikido, this bow happens inside. You bow to the anger that taught you boundaries. You bow to the fear that kept you alert. You bow to the sadness that opened your empathy. The bow means: "I honor your message. You can rest now". It is the ritual of closure that turns raw emotion into wisdom.

6.10 The Lesson of the Chapter

To be welcome is to transform emotion from invader to ally. It's the third gate of Emotional Aikido —the bridge between awareness and compassion. Every feeling, once welcomed, changes its shape.

Anger becomes courage. Fear becomes attention. Sadness becomes depth. Guilt becomes integrity. The emotional aikidoka knows that no emotion is against him. Each is a teacher disguised as tension, a visitor that comes to restore wholeness.

When you stop running from what you feel, you stop running from yourself. And only then can peace truly begin.

CHAPTER 7.
Benevolence: responding with Empathy and Inner Strength

7.1 The Silent Power of Conscious Kindness

To be benevolent is not to be weak. It is to have enough strength to remain calm in chaos, and enough clarity not to mirror the energy that hurts you. **Benevolence** is the art of keeping the heart open when everything invites it to close.

Modern society often confuses empathy with fragility and kindness with submission. Yet neuroscience reveals that compassion activates the brain's most evolved regions —those linked to morality, purpose, and creativity.

Benevolence is not a soft emotion; it is a **regulatory force** — the point where Emotional Aikido becomes visible in action. To practice benevolence does not mean allowing abuse. It means responding without losing dignity.

The emotional aikidoka does not react to win arguments; he acts to restore balance. His goal is not victory, but elevation of consciousness.

7.2 The Neurobiology of Active Compassion

• The benevolent brain operates differently.

When we experience genuine empathy and compassion, specific neural circuits light up:

• The **ventromedial prefrontal cortex**, integrating emotion and morality.

• The **anterior insula**, allowing us to feel what others feel without losing center.

• The **oxytocin system**, fostering trust and cooperation.

• The **vagus nerve**, regulating calm, tone of voice, and social engagement.

From a physiological perspective, benevolence is a state of coherence between body, emotion, and thought.

It is not mere sympathy —it is **synchronicity** between one nervous system and another. That is why one calm person can pacify an entire group; their nervous system emits safety signals that others unconsciously mirror. Benevolence literally **reshapes the emotional field around us**.

7.3 From Empathy to Equilibrium

Emotional empathy means feeling what another feels; benevolence means **feeling without losing yourself**.

The balance lies in accompanying without absorbing, helping without carrying, understanding without merging. Many caregivers, therapists, and leaders suffer from compassion fatigue —empathy without grounding.

Benevolence offers the antidote: a compassionate presence anchored in self-regulation.

A simple mantra summarizes this balance: "I can be with your pain without losing my peace". That is benevolence —love that understands yet remains strong.

7.4 Exercise 1: benevolent Breathing (3 minutes)

1- Close your eyes. Inhale slowly through your nose, thinking: "I receive calm".

2- Exhale softly through your mouth, thinking: "I send calm".

3- Repeat for three minutes, imagining each breath connecting you with the well-being of others.

4- If someone comes to mind, visualize your exhalation surrounding them with serenity —without needing to change them.

This exercise trains the brain to modulate empathy with stability. It activates the vagus nerve and strengthens parasympathetic tone —biological foundations of compassion.

7.5 Exercise 2: the Aikidoka Response

When someone attacks or provokes you, remember the three steps of the aikidoka:

1- **Breathe before responding:** Regulate before defending.

2- **Acknowledge the other's emotion:** "I can see you're upset".

3- **Respond from center:** steady voice, calm eyes, balanced posture.

Such a response deactivates the other person's amygdala and shifts the conflict dynamic. It's not submission —it's conscious strategy. Instead of mirroring aggression, you neutralize it through presence.

7.6 Benevolence as Strategic Intelligence

In martial Aikido, rigidity breaks you; fluidity saves you. The same applies emotionally: if you respond with hardness, you amplify harm; with calm, you transform energy. Benevolence does not deny conflict—it **redirects** it. Neurologically, it shifts the response pathway from the sympathetic (defensive) to the parasympathetic (regulatory) system. Spiritually, it turns reaction into wisdom.

7.7 The Paradox of Soft Power

Benevolence is the highest form of power —the kind that transforms without imposing. From Gandhi's nonviolent resistance to the therapist's calm in crisis, history shows that compassionate leadership achieves deeper, longer-lasting change.

Aggressive power conquers territories; benevolent power conquers hearts.

And in the long run, it is the heart that governs destiny.

7.8 Exercise 3: the Circle of Gratitude

Each night, before sleeping, write down three acts of benevolence you offered or witnessed:

- A kind word that shifted the mood.
- A moment of patience that prevented conflict.
- A smile that lightened someone's burden.

Then write one sentence: "Today, I chose to respond instead of react".

This simple ritual reinforces the neural circuits of gratitude and moral serenity.

7.9 Benevolence and Healthy Boundaries

To be benevolent does not mean saying yes to everything.

Saying **no** peacefully is also an act of compassion. The emotional aikidoka sets boundaries without violence—protecting energy while keeping the heart open.

A benevolent boundary says: "I won't let you harm me, but I wish you no harm". That is the sacred frontier between empathy and self-respect.

7.10 The Lesson of the Chapter

Benevolence is the fourth gate of Emotional Aikido. If anticipate means perceiving, analyze means understanding, and be welcome means accepting, then benevolence means **responding**

from wisdom. It is the union of love and firmness, empathy and clarity. It turns impulse into intention and emotion into conscious action.

The emotional aikidoka does not seek to be right —he seeks to be at peace. He knows that every true victory begins within. And that benevolence, far from weakness, is the highest expression of human strength.

CHAPTER 8.
Control: mastering the Body, Breath, and Mental Focus

8.1 The Discipline of Inner Stability

Control is not repression—it is direction. It is the art of guiding the storm without denying that the wind exists. True control in Emotional Aikido is not about silencing emotion, but about channeling it through awareness, posture, and breath until chaos turns into clarity.

Most people think of control as tension: clenched fists, held breath, forced calm. But authentic control feels the opposite —it is **fluid, alert, and centered**.

The aikidoka knows that mastery does not come from rigidity, but from presence.

He becomes the eye of the hurricane: still, observing, unmovable inside. Control, in its highest form, is **freedom from automatic reaction**.

8.2 The Neurophysiology of Self-Regulation

To control emotion is to regulate the nervous system. Every emotional reaction starts as a physiological wave—a rise in heart rate, a shift in breathing, a surge of adrenaline. The **vagus nerve**, running from the brainstem to the heart and gut, is the main conductor of calm. When it is activated, it slows the heartbeat, lowers blood pressure, and rebalances the body's chemistry. This process, called **vagal tone**, determines how quickly you can return to serenity after stress. High vagal tone equals resilience. Low vagal tone equals vulnerability to anxiety, anger, and fatigue. Training control, therefore, means **training the vagus nerve** —through breath, posture, and focus.

8.3 Breath: the Bridge Between Mind and Body

Breathing is the only physiological function we can consciously regulate that immediately alters emotional states. Fast, shallow breathing triggers the sympathetic system (fight or flight). Slow, deep breathing activates the parasympathetic system (rest and restore).

In Aikido, the concept of **Kokyu** means "breath of harmony". In Emotional Aikido, it is the same: to breathe in rhythm with what is happening instead of fighting against it. **Controlled breathing transforms energy**. When you breathe deeply, you're not escaping emotion—you're giving it space to reorganize.

8.4 Exercise 1: centering Breath (The Three Circles)

1- Sit or stand upright, feet grounded.

2- Inhale through your nose for 4 seconds, expanding your abdomen.

3- Hold your breath for 2 seconds, feeling stability.

4- Exhale through your mouth for 6 seconds, softening your shoulders.

5- Visualize three circles aligning—your head (thought), heart (emotion), and abdomen (instinct).

Repeat three times, noticing how your pulse slows and clarity returns. This exercise builds the neurophysiological habit of calm focus—essential for emotional mastery.

8.5 The Posture of the Center (Hara)

In Japanese philosophy, the **Hara** —the area two fingers below the navel— is the center of gravity and energy. When you lose emotional control, your energy rises to your head; thoughts spin, voice tightens, heart races. To regain control, bring awareness back to the Hara.

Try this:

- Stand tall.
- Place your hand on your lower abdomen.
- Inhale into that space, feeling weight and grounding.
- Imagine roots descending from your feet into the earth.

The more grounded your body, the calmer your mind. The brain reads posture as feedback: when you stabilize the body, you stabilize the mind.

8.6 The Science of Focus (Attentional Control)

Emotional regulation depends on attention regulation. When your focus is scattered, emotions dominate; when you focus consciously, you become the observer, not the reactor. The **dorsolateral prefrontal cortex** is the region that maintains attention on what truly matters.

Meditation, mindfulness, and breath work strengthen this region like a muscle.

Repeated practice rewires your brain to return to center faster after emotional turbulence. Every focused breath is a micro-rehearsal of self-command.

8.7 Exercise 2: the Five-Second Reset

Whenever you feel overwhelmed:

1- Pause whatever you're doing.

2- Inhale for **five seconds.**

3- Exhale for **five seconds.**

4- While exhaling, think: "I am returning to center".

This small ritual sends a direct signal to the vagus nerve, instantly slowing the body's stress response. It's the aikidoka's invisible technique —subtle yet powerful.

8.8 Emotional Control vs. Suppression

Suppression is holding your breath under water; control is learning to swim. Suppression stores tension in the body, which later appears as fatigue, headaches, or even chronic illness. Control, in contrast, allows the wave to move through you without drowning in it. Emotional control is not about silence —it's about rhythm. It's knowing when to speak, when to breathe, and when to let go.

8.9 The Triad of Mastery: Breath, Body and Mind

Emotional control emerges when these three systems synchronize:

Element	Function	Practice
Breath	Regulates the nervous system	Slow, rhythmic breathing (4-2-6)
Body	Anchors attention and presence	Postural awareness, grounding
Mind	Directs and interprets	Mindful observation, focus on Hara

When these three align, emotion becomes energy under direction—not under domination. This is the state that Aikido masters call Shin-Tai-Ichi —the unity of mind, body, and spirit.

8.10 The Lesson of the Chapter

Control is the fifth gate of Emotional Aikido. It is the art of holding yourself together when the world around you begins to scatter. To control is not to avoid intensity, but to **inhabit** it consciously. It is to breathe while others hold their breath, to stand firm while others fall into reaction. The emotional aikidoka does not need to shout, argue, or flee. His control is quiet yet magnetic.

He radiates stability —the kind that comes from deep breath, grounded presence and mental focus. That calm becomes his most persuasive force. Because the one who masters himself, masters the moment.

CHAPTER 9.
Change: breaking Patterns and Reprogramming Thought

9.1 The Invisible Movement of Inner Transformation

Change is not about becoming someone else —it is about **returning to who you are without the weight of fear**. True change does not come from external pressure; it rises from within, when awareness illuminates what was once automatic. Most people want to change their emotions without changing their habits of thought. But the brain doesn't transform what it merely understands —it transforms what it **practices**.

That's why, in Emotional Aikido, change is active, embodied, and repetitive: a dance between the mind that observes, the body that learns, and the soul that releases. Every repeated emotion carves a neural groove; every repeated thought reinforces a circuit.

To change is to **retrain those pathways** —not by force, but through consistency, consciousness, and compassion.

9.2 Neuroplasticity: the Biological Art of Reinvention

The brain is malleable, even in adulthood. Each time you choose a new emotional response, you are literally **redrawing**

your neural map. Science calls this **neuroplasticity** —the brain's ability to create, strengthen or weaken connections based on experience.

When you repeat an emotional habit —worry, guilt, fear— the associated synapses grow stronger. But when you introduce a new conscious response —breathing, observing, reframing— the brain builds an alternative circuit.

Through repetition, that new pathway becomes faster, stronger, more natural. Change, therefore, doesn't happen through sudden enlightenment but through **lucid repetition**. Every act of awareness is a sculptor's strike on the architecture of your brain.

9.3 From Automatic Thought to Conscious Thought

Ninety percent of the thoughts you have today are the same ones you had yesterday. Change begins the moment you interrupt that automatic loop, even for a single second.

The emotional aikidoka breaks the pattern with one question: "Does this thought serve me, or does it chain me?" That brief pause changes everything. The amygdala loosens its grip, and the prefrontal cortex regains control. You stop being a reaction and become a decision.

Change is not suppressing what you feel —it is **reinterpreting** what it means to feel.

It is not eliminating pain —it is discovering its purpose. It is not denying fear —it is transforming it into prudence.

9.4 The Formula of Microchanges (Two Minutes a Day)

The brain loves repetition, not drastic leaps. That's why the Emotional Aikido method teaches **microchanges** —small, sustainable shifts that reprogram without resistance.

Examples:

• Instead of promising "I won't get angry again", decide to **observe your anger for two minutes before acting.**

- Instead of saying "I'll be positive", decide to **find one neutral thought** when a negative one appears.
- Instead of "I'm going to change my life", start with **one conscious breath each morning**.
- Big transformations begin with micro-movements. Lasting change doesn't come from force, but from **gentle consistency**.

9.5 Exercise 1: cognitive Reframing (The Art of Reinterpretation)

1- Identify a recurring emotion or thought.

2- Write it down as a short statement: "I feel ______________ because ____".

3- Add a second statement that opens a new perspective: "It could also mean that ____".

Example:

"I feel afraid because things are changing".

"It could also mean that I'm growing and my mind just hasn't adapted yet".

This reframing activates the **dorsolateral prefrontal cortex**, the brain region responsible for generating new interpretations and breaking rigid thought patterns.

9.6 Exercise 2: reverse Visualization (Mental Aikido)

Phyical Aikido teaches us to redirect the opponent's energy. Emotionally, we can do the same with negative thoughts.

1- Close your eyes and visualize the emotion as a stream of energy approaching you.

2- Instead of blocking it, imagine yourself turning with it in a circular motion, like in an Aikido technique.

3- See the energy losing force as it flows.

4- End by imagining that energy transforming into light or clarity.

This is not fantasy —it is neural training.
You are teaching the brain to **reinterpret stimulus as information, not as threat.**

9.7 Breaking the Cycle of Self-Criticism

Nothing blocks change more than judgment. Every time you say "I'll never change", you're strengthening the neural pattern of stagnation. Change requires observation, not condemnation.

Repeat this mantra: "I'm learning. I didn't fail—I'm practicing". The brain learns through compassion, not punishment. Every mistake is data, not defeat.

9.8 The Power of Conscious Emotional Habit

Emotional habits are the bridge between mind and body. When an emotion repeats, the body remembers it before the mind does. Thus, change means **retraining sensations**, not just thoughts.

Each time you practice calm, even if you don't feel it completely, your body memorizes it. Each time you choose to breathe instead of shout, your nervous system learns a new survival route.

Over time, emotional control stops being effort and becomes **a bodily memory of serenity**.

9.9 The Circle of Conscious Change

The Emotional Aikido process of transformation follows this sequence:

1- **Perceive (Anticipate):** notice the emotion before the impulse.
2- **Understand (Analyze):** find its meaning.
3- **Accept (Be welcome):** make space for it.
4- **Respond (Benevolence):** act with calm and empathy.
5- **Direct (Control):** regulate body and mind.
6- **Reprogram (Change):** create a new neural path.

The cycle doesn't close through force —it closes through awareness. Each round strengthens the next, forming an upward spiral of inner evolution.

9.10 The Lesson of the Chapter

Change is the sixth gate of Emotional Aikido.

It is not an event —it is a training. Change does not happen when you say, "I want to change," but when your breath, your body, and your mind learn to move together.

To change is to dance with life without clinging to the past. To trust that every emotion carries a meaning, and that by integrating it, you become freer. To realize that every new thought is an opportunity to be reborn.

The emotional aikidoka does not seek perfection —he seeks awareness. And in that awareness, he discovers that real change is not forward or backward, but **inward**.

CHAPTER 10.
Defeat: deactivating Toxic Cycles whithout Destroying the Other

10.1 The True Art of Victory

In traditional Aikido, victory does not mean overpowering the opponent—it means dissolving the conflict before harm occurs. The same principle guides **Emotional Aikido:** to win without wounding, to neutralize the cycle of negativity while preserving dignity—both yours and the other's.

The emotional aikidoka understands that **every conflict is an energy loop:** one person attacks, the other reacts, the first one defends, and so on. Breaking the cycle doesn't come from dominance, but from awareness. To defeat in this context means to **disarm violence**, **not through force**, **but through consciousness**. True victory is peace restored, not ego satisfied.

10.2 The Anatomy of a Toxic Cycle

Every toxic exchange follows a predictable pattern:

1- Trigger: Something ignites emotional tension.

2- Reaction: You feel attacked, criticized, or invalidated.

3- Escalation: The nervous system prepares for combat.

4- Repetition: Old wounds and patterns replay themselves.

5- Exhaustion: Both sides feel drained, misunderstood, defeated.

This is not just psychology —it's neurobiology. The **amygdala** interprets threat, floods the system with adrenaline, and silences the rational mind.

If neither person regulates the surge, both become reactive mirrors —amplifying the same pain. To defeat the cycle, you must step **outside the mirror**. You don't fight the reflection —you calm the one reflected.

10.3 The Warrior of Consciousness

In Emotional Aikido, the warrior does not conquer others; he conquers his **reactions**. He transforms the energy of anger into clarity, the impulse to attack into the power to pause. He recognizes that the most dangerous battlefield is the mind that refuses to understand.

To defeat without destroying is to **convert emotion into intelligence**. It is to see conflict as an invitation to grow, not a proof of who is right. It is to learn the sacred paradox: you can stop a fight by refusing to participate in it unconsciously.

10.4 Exercise 1: the Pause That Disarms

When you sense a conflict escalating, practice the **Three-Breath Rule:**

1- First breath: Feel your body—heart, muscles, jaw. Don't speak.

2- Second breath: Notice your emotion—anger, fear, sadness. Don't analyze.

3- Third breath: Ask yourself, "What's needed here: reaction or resolution?"

Then respond, not from the wound, but from the center.

This simple technique gives the prefrontal cortex time to regain control, lowering cortisol and calming the vagus nerve. You stop being the echo and become the anchor.

10.5 The Triangle of Drama and How to Dissolve It

Psychologist Stephen Karpman described three unconscious roles that perpetuate emotional suffering:

- **Victim:** "Poor me".
- **Persecutor:** "It's your fault".
- **Rescuer:** "I'll fix you".

These roles rotate endlessly in families, relationships and workplaces. The antidote is **conscious neutrality:** stepping out of the triangle entirely. The aikidoka emotional mantra is: "I choose not to play this role. I choose awareness instead". This breaks the pattern of projection and opens the door to authentic connection.

10.6 The Power of De-escalation

Conflict is fire. Every reaction either feeds it or extinguishes it. De-escalation is not weakness —it's mastery of emotional chemistry. To de-escalate, apply the **Four Movements of the Inner Aikido:**

1- **Lower your voice:** activates calm in the listener's vagus nerve.

2- **Slow your breath:** signals safety to both nervous systems.

3- **Soften your posture:** communicates openness, not submission.

4- **Speak from "I":** transforms accusation into authenticity.

Example: instead of "You never listen," say "I feel unheard when this happens". Language is energy. Change the phrasing, and you change the physiology of the conversation.

10.7 Exercise 2: compassionate Boundaries

Write a list of situations or people where conflict drains your peace. For each, practice defining a **benevolent boundary:**

Situation	Old Reaction	New Conscious Response
Criticism	Defend or attack	"I hear your point. Let me reflect on it".
Manipulation	Give in or withdraw	"I value honesty; let's speak openly".
Shouting	Raise voice	"I'll talk when we're both calm".

Boundaries are not walls —they are **frames of respect**. They teach others how to meet your presence without invading it.

10.8 Dissolving the Inner Enemy

Every external conflict mirrors an internal one. We cannot end hostility outside until we reconcile it within. Often, the person we are trying to defeat represents a part of ourselves that we have rejected.

Ask yourself: "What part of me reacts like this? What am I defending so fiercely?" The answer reveals the real battlefield: between your current self and the self still trapped in old pain. The moment you see this, the opponent loses power —because you have found the lesson.

10.9 The Evolution of Conflict into Wisdom

Every clash is an invitation to maturity. The higher self uses tension as a sculptor uses friction —to polish the rough edges of ego. When you meet aggression with clarity and compassion, you are no longer playing the same game. You stop perpetuating karma and begin practicing **Dharma:** conscious action aligned with purpose. You transform energy instead of transmitting it.

10.10 The Lesson of the Chapter

Defeat is the seventh gate of Emotional Aikido. It is not about crushing the opponent, but **breaking the cycle of unconscious reaction**. The emotional aikidoka no longer fights against life; **he dances with it**.

He learns that peace is not the absence of conflict, but the ability to stay centered within it. He disarms not with power, but with presence. He defeats not through victory, but through understanding. Because the ultimate opponent is never the other person— it is the part of ourselves that still believes we must fight to prove we exist.

CHAPTER 11.
Dissolve: closing, Cleansing, and Releasing Emotional Load

11.1 The Art of Letting Go Without Losing the Lesson

To dissolve is not to forget. It is to **release without erasing**. It is allowing emotion to complete its natural cycle so that the mind and body can return to balance.

In **Emotional Aikido**, dissolving represents the final movement —the moment when energy stops being conflict and becomes understanding. Everything that is not dissolved becomes residue.

Unexpressed emotions do not vanish; they settle in the body—hidden in the muscles, the stomach, or the chest. Tension is undigested memory. To dissolve is to allow that trapped energy to exhale, melt, and finally be set free.

The emotional aikidoka knows the battle ends when the breath returns to its natural rhythm. That exhalation —the deep sigh after conflict— is the true victory.

11.2 The Neurochemistry of Emotional Closure

Every emotion follows a biological cycle. It begins with **activation** (adrenaline, cortisol, increased heart rate), continues with

expression (through action or thought), and ends with **resolution** (oxytocin, serotonin, calm).

When the cycle is not completed, the nervous system remains in alert mode. That's why many people sleep but never rest, forgive but never feel free. Their body is still "holding the sword".

Dissolving activates the **recovery system:**

• **Oxytocin** restores connection and tenderness.

• **Serotonin** stabilizes mood.

• **Acetylcholine** slows the stress response.

• The **vagus nerve** brings harmony back between heart and breath.

The biology of forgiveness exists —it is called **homeostatic restoration**.

11.3 The Complete Emotional Cycle

1- **Perceive** the emotion.

2- **Name** it without judgment.

3- **Breathe** through it to allow expression.

4- **Listen** to understand its message.

5- **Release** it with gratitude.

Without the final step —letting go— the process remains incomplete. Emotion needs recognition, not imprisonment.

11.4 Exercise 1: the Dissolving Breath (5 minutes)

1- Sit in silence.

2- Close your eyes and visualize the emotion still present in you.

3- Inhale deeply through your nose, imagining you're drawing in clarity.

4- Exhale slowly through your mouth, visualizing a gray mist leaving your body.

5- With each exhale, repeat silently: "I release you. Thank you for what you taught me".

This practice trains the nervous system to close emotional cycles without repression. It is a physical form of **forgiveness through the body**, not just through the mind.

11.5 Exercise 2: the Ritual of Closure (Therapeutic Writing)

Take a sheet of paper and write a letter to the emotion, person, or situation that still weighs on you. Not to send, but to **free yourself**.

Include three parts:

1- **Recognition:** "This is what I lived and how I felt".

2- **Gratitude:** "Thank you for what you showed me, even if it hurt".

3- **Release:** "I no longer need to carry this. I let you go".

After writing, tear, burn, or keep the paper —whatever feels right to your intuition. This symbolic act completes the **neurological circuit of closure**.

11.6 Silence as Emotional Medicine

Noise keeps thoughts alive; silence transforms them. In silence, the brain enters a coherent state—alpha and theta waves emerge, allowing emotional integration.

The emotional aikidoka learns that silence is not emptiness — it is **psychic digestion space**· It's in silence that the soul organizes what it has learned. After a conflict, the greatest act of wisdom is not always to speak, but to **breathe and let the body finish the dialogue**.

11.7 Compassion as the Universal Solvent

Nothing dissolves resentment faster than compassion —not only toward others, but toward oneself. Compassion doesn't justify what happened, but it **breaks identification with the wound**.

It reminds you that you can have suffered without becoming your suffering. When you whisper inwardly, “May all beings — including myself— be at peace”, something shifts in your body chemistry.

The amygdala calms. The breath expands. The heart softens. Not because the past has changed, but because **you no longer hold it from the wound, but from awareness.**

11.8 Exercise 3: the Minute of Integration

At the end of each day, sit in silence for one minute and ask yourself:

- What emotion needs closure today?
- What can I release that no longer serves me?
- What did I learn from what hurt me?

Do not force answers —just feel. This daily minute prevents emotional residue and trains the brain to complete its cycles naturally.

11.9 Dissolution as a Spiritual Principle

To dissolve is not to lose —it is to **reunite**. In nature, everything that disintegrates gives birth to something new. The river doesn't fight the rock; it shapes it into art.

Likewise, the emotional aikidoka doesn't destroy emotion — he transforms it into wisdom. Every tear that falls, every anger that softens, every fear that dissolves leaves behind a new clarity. The ego fears dissolution because it confuses permanence with existence. But the soul knows that to dissolve is to **return to the flow of life itself**.

11.10 The Lesson of the Chapter

Dissolve is the eighth and final gate of Emotional Aikido. It completes the cycle of the **2A + 2B + 2C + 2D system:** anticipate, analyze, be welcome, benevolence, control, change, defeat, and dissolve.

To dissolve is **the final alchemy** —the transformation of conflict into consciousness.

When emotion dissolves, it doesn't disappear —it integrates. When a wound closes, it doesn't vanish —it becomes wisdom. The emotional aikidoka knows that life is not about conquering —it's about **releasing**.

Because only when the heart lets go can the soul truly breathe again. And in that last conscious exhalation, the cycle completes itself: the mind rests, the body lightens, and peace ceases to be a goal —it becomes **our natural state**.

PART III.
Emotional Aikido Protocols for Everyday Life

CHAPTER 12.
Protocols of emotional Aikido in daily life

12.1 The Bridge between Inner Harmony and Outer Action

Emotional Aikido is not a philosophy to be admired —it is a discipline to be lived. Its true mastery is revealed not in silence, but in the chaos of ordinary life: in the argument with a loved one, in the tension of leadership, in the uncertainty of illness, in the fatigue of caregiving.

Wherever human emotion arises, the art applies. Each of the eight principles —Anticipate, Analyze, Be welcome, Benevolence, Control, Change, Defeat, and Dissolve— becomes a compass, helping you transform reactivity into conscious action. The dojo of Emotional Aikido is not a mat —it is your everyday existence.

12.2 Application 1. Personal Relationships: turning Conflict into Connection

Relationships are emotional mirrors. They reflect both our love and our unhealed parts. When two nervous systems meet, they can either harmonize or collide.

In moments of conflict, the aikidoka applies this sequence:

1- **Anticipate:** Sense the tension before words appear. Watch for body cues—breath, tone, gaze.

2- **Analyze:** Identify the real emotion behind the reaction. (Anger often hides hurt).

3- **Be welcome:** Allow the feeling in yourself and the other. Acceptance precedes understanding.

4- **Benevolence:** Respond from kindness, not defense.

5- **Control:** Ground your body and slow your voice.

6- **Change:** Reframe the dialogue. "It's not you vs. me —it's us vs. the problem".

7- **Defeat:** Deactivate escalation; don't feed the cycle.

8- **Dissolve:** Close the exchange with gratitude and silence.

Love is not sustained by perfect communication, but by **conscious repair**. Emotional Aikido teaches that harmony is not the absence of friction —it is the art of returning to it gracefully.

12.3 Application 2. Leadership and Work: calm Amidst Complexity

In organizations, emotional contagion spreads faster than information. A single regulated leader can stabilize an entire team. The leader trained in Emotional Aikido does not command by control, but by **coherence**. His calm nervous system becomes a tuning fork for those around him. He listens before he acts, redirects tension with empathy, and responds from intention rather than impulse. **Practical Microtechniques for the Workplace:**

1- Begin meetings with 30 seconds of collective silence or breathing.

2- Replace "Who's to blame?" with "What is needed now?"

3- When under pressure, lower your tone instead of raising it.

4- Offer feedback through the 3A principle: **Acknowledge, Ask, Align**.

Leadership rooted in Aikido is not dominance —it is **direction through presence**.

12.4 Application 3. Medicine and Mental Healdth: The Healing Power of Regulation

In therapy, psychiatry, and caregiving, Emotional Aikido becomes a clinical tool.

When a professional is centered, patients regulate through resonance—a phenomenon known as **co-regulation**.

A psychiatrist practicing Emotional Aikido:

- Anticipates emotional storms before they appear.
- Uses benevolence instead of authority to calm anxiety.
- Controls his own physiology to model safety.
- Changes the energy of the session with tone, silence or humor.
- Dissolves transference through compassion and neutrality.

Healing, at its core, is **energetic alignment** between two nervous systems. When the clinician embodies coherence, the patient's biology learns what peace feels like.

12.5 Application 4. Parenting and Education: teaching Children Emotional Flow

Children don't learn emotional intelligence through words, but through imitation. They absorb the rhythm of our nervous system long before they understand language.

Applying Aikido at home means:

- Anticipating tantrums by noticing early tension.
- Analyzing emotions rather than labeling behavior. ("You're angry" instead of "You're bad").
- Welcoming tears as release, not rebellion.
- Showing benevolence by staying near, not by fixing.
- Controlling your own breathing to model calm.
- Changing routines that overstimulate.
- Defeating chaos by soft tone and structure.
- Dissolving tension through touch, silence, or humor.

To raise emotionally intelligent children, we must first become emotionally **regulated adults**.

12.6 Application 5: crisis and Conflict Management

When life hits hard—loss, betrayal, failure —the reflex is to tighten. Aikido teaches the opposite: **enter, blend, redirect**. In crisis, the eight principles become survival tools:

- **Anticipate:** Recognize early signs of overwhelm.
- **Analyze:** Identify needs beneath fear.
- **Be welcome:** Allow emotion to pass through.
- **Benevolence:** Treat yourself gently.
- **Control:** Anchor the body—sit, breathe, stay.
- **Change:** Adjust expectations to reality.
- **Defeat:** Stop feeding self-destructive cycles.
- **Dissolve:** Let the storm end before acting again.

Resilience is not toughness—it is flexibility under pressure. Emotional Aikido restores that flexibility, both physiologically and spiritually.

12.7 Guided Exercise: the Daily Aikido Practice (10 minutes)

1- **Morning (2 min):** Breath alignment: inhale calm, exhale clarity.

2- **Midday (2 min):** Grounding pause: check posture, soften shoulders, reset.

3- **Evening (3 min):** Emotional reflection: what emotion dominated today?

4- **Night (3 min):** Dissolving breath: release tension, bless the day, rest.

In ten minutes, you train your nervous system to reset itself. Over time, your baseline becomes calm rather than chaos.

12.8 The Lesson of the Chapter

The world doesn't need more control —it needs **more coherence**. Emotional Aikido invites us to respond to modern chaos with ancient balance. Its wisdom lies not in fighting emotion, but in flowing with it consciously.

Wherever there is tension, there is potential for practice. Every argument, every challenge, every difficult moment becomes a **dojo for the soul**. Because the true master of Emotional Aikido is not the one who avoids conflict, but the one who turns it into compassion in real time.

CHAPTER 13.
Twelve-Week Emotional Training Program

A practical manual to integrate the eight disciplines of Emotional Aikido (2A + 2B + 2C + 2D)

13.1 Introduction: From Knowledge to Daily Practice

Theory becomes wisdom only when it is embodied. The **12-Week Emotional Aikido Program** was designed to transform the eight principles —Anticipate, Analyze, Be welcome, Benevolence, Control, Change, Defeat, and Dissolve— into neural, emotional, and behavioral habits.

Each week develops a specific dimension of emotional consciousness through breathing, reflection, journaling, movement, and mindful interaction. The goal is not to change what you feel, but **how you relate to what you feel**.

Twelve weeks are enough for the brain, body, and mind to begin working in a new emotional rhythm—more conscious, more coherent, more serene.

13.2 Program Structure

Duration: 12 weeks

Daily practice: 2–3 short sessions (morning, afternoon, night).

Practice length: 10–15 minutes.

Tools: an emotional journal, a quiet space, and consistency.

Each week includes:

- One **core principle** (from the 2A + 2B + 2C + 2D system).
- A clear **emotional goal**.
- **Guided exercises**.
- A **reflective question**.
- A **microhabit plan** for continuity.

WEEK 1: ANTICIPATE: ACTIVATING THE RADAR OF AWARENESS

Goal: Learn to recognize emotional signals before they escalate.

Exercises:

- Morning body scan (3 minutes).
- "Micro-signal log": write down three moments when you noticed tension without reacting.
- Emotional traffic light: stop, observe, breathe before speaking.

Reflection: What patterns always begin before my conflicts?

WEEK 2: ANALYZE: UNDERSTANDING THE MESSAGE BEHIND EMOTION

Goal: Translate emotion into meaningful information.

Exercises:

- Emotion journal with three columns: situation/emotion/unmet need.
- The "Three Causes" method: What triggered it? What sustains it? What can I learn?
- Cognitive reframing of one recurring thought.

Reflection: What am I really trying to protect each time I react?

WEEK 3: WELCOME: TURNING EMOTION INTO AN ALLY

Goal: Learn to feel without fleeing.

Exercises:

- Morning "welcoming breath" (2 minutes).
- Internal dialogue with the dominant emotion of the day.
- "Inner Guest" meditation: visualize emotion as a temporary visitor.

Reflection: What changes when I stop resisting what I feel?

WEEK 4: BENEVOLENCE: RESPONDING WITH EMPATHY AND INNER STRENGTH

Goal: Act with compassion without losing firmness.

Exercises:

- Benevolent breathing (inhale calm, exhale understanding).
- Mirror compassion exercise: speak kindly to yourself out loud.
- Daily gratitude and nonviolent communication practice.

Reflection: What happens when I choose to respond rather than react?

WEEK 5: CONTROL: MASTERING BODY, BREATH, AND FOCUS

Goal: Learn to regulate your nervous system in real time.

Exercises:

- 4-2-6 breathing three times daily.
- Centering posture (Hara) before stressful events.
- Five seconds reset: a short pause amid chaos.

Reflection: Which part of my body warns me first when I lose center?

WEEK 6: CHANGE: REPROGRAMMING PATTERNS AND REACTIONS

Goal: Break automatic emotional loops.

Exercises:

- One microchange per day: a new response to an old emotion.

• Reverse visualization: redirect negative thoughts like circular energy.

• Progress journal: record even small advances.

Reflection: What emotional habit am I ready to transform this week?

WEEK 7: DEFEAT: BREAKING TOXIC CYCLES WITHOUT DAMAGE

Goal: Stop reactivity without destroying connection.

Exercises:

• The three-breath rule before responding to conflict.

• Write compassionate boundaries for difficult people.

• Identify where you play the "drama triangle" (victim, persecutor, rescuer).

Reflection: What do I gain when I choose peace over being right?

WEEK 8: DISSOLVE: RELEASING AND COMPLETING THE EMOTIONAL CYCLE

Goal: Learn to close and let go with gratitude.

Exercises:

• Dissolving breath (5 minutes before sleep).

• Write a letter of closure to an emotion, person, or past situation.

• One-minute integration: notice what emotion needs to be released today.

Reflection: How does my body feel once an emotion is fully dissolved?

WEEK 9: INTEGRATING THE FULL FLOW (2A + 2B + 2C + 2D)

Goal: Unite the eight gates into one conscious flow.

Exercises:

• Emotional circle practice: mentally walk through all eight principles during a real conflict.

• Integrative breathing (eight deep cycles, one for each principle).

• Observation log: document one real-life experience using the full method.

Reflection: How does my energy shift when I apply the full Aikido sequence?

WEEK 10: THE BODY AS TEACHER

Goal: Strengthen interoception and body-mind coherence.

Exercises:

• Gentle body scan with music.

• Record daily physical sensations linked to emotion.

• Free movement practice: let your body express without judgment.

Reflection: Where does calm live in my body? Where does tension hide?

WEEK 11: RELATIONSHIP AS DOJO

Goal: Apply Emotional Aikido in human connection.

Exercises:

• Conscious conversation: listen without interrupting or preparing answers.

• De-escalation practice: turn disagreement into understanding.

• Benevolence-in-action: respond calmly to criticism.

Reflection: What have I learned about myself through my reactions to others?

WEEK 12: LIVING IN THE AIKIDO STATE

Goal: Consolidate the practice and turn it into a lifestyle.

Exercises:

• Master breathing (8 minutes integrating all principles).

• Emotional maintenance plan: design your own rituals of serenity.

• Letter to your future self: "This is what harmony feels like".

Reflection: Who am I now that I've completed this inner training?

13.3 Long-Term Recommendations for Coherence

- **Practice even when you don't need it:** serenity is trained before the storm.
- Don't seek results, seek **rhythm**.
- Celebrate small victories: a single conscious breath counts.
- Remember: **Emotional Aikido doesn't end at Week 12**, it begins each day you choose awareness over reaction.

13.4 Closing of the Program

The goal is not to control life, but to **move with it**. Every breath, every pause, every act of kindness is Aikido in motion. After twelve weeks, you will not have learned to avoid conflict—you will have learned to **transform it into consciousness**. And once that happens, you no longer practice Emotional Aikido, **you embody it**.

PART IV.
Scientific and Practical Bases of Emotional Aikido

CHAPTER 14.
Aikido-IE Questionnaire (Aikido Emotional Intelligence Appraisal)

A comprehensive emotional assessment tool based on the 2A + 2B + 2C + 2D Emotional Aikido System

14.1 General Introduction

The **Aikido-IE (Aikido Emotional Intelligence Appraisal)** is a 24-item self-assessment designed to evaluate an individual's ability to perceive, regulate, and transform emotions through the eight disciplines of the **2A + 2B + 2C + 2D Emotional Aikido System: Anticipate, Analyze, Welcome, Benevolence, Control, Change, Defeat and Dissolve.**

Unlike traditional emotional intelligence tests that focus mainly on perception or social interaction, the Aikido-IE measures one's capacity to **transform emotional energy into psychophysiological coherence** —to convert reaction into presence, and resistance into flow.

It integrates **neuroscience, clinical psychology, and Eastern philosophy** providing a structured way to identify both **strengths and blockages** in emotional processing and regulation.

14.2 Theoretical Foundations

Each of the eight principles corresponds to three interrelated levels of functioning:

1- **Physiological level:** how the body reacts to emotional stimuli (heart rate, breathing, muscle tone).

2- **Cognitive level:** how the emotion is interpreted (automatic thoughts, beliefs, narrative).

3- **Behavioral level:** how the person responds (impulsivity, control, compassion, repair).

The Aikido-IE measures these through 24 short statements —three per domain— creating an **eight-dimensional emotional profile** that reflects balance and integration.

14.3 Administration Guidelines

- **Target population:** adults and adolescents (16 years or older)
- **Completion time:** 8–10 minutes
- **Format:** self-report, paper or digital.
- **Response scale:**

  1 = Almost never.

  2 = Rarely.

  3 = Sometimes.

  4 = Often.

  5 = Almost always.

Participants are instructed to answer based on **how they actually respond in life**, not how they wish they would respond. The test should be completed in a calm, private space, ideally after a few deep breaths.

14.4 Instrument Structure

Code	Principle	Brief Definition	Emotional Objective
A1–A3	Anticipate	Detect internal and external signals before escalation.	Prevent impulsive reaction.
A4–A6	Analyze	Understand the cause and message of emotions.	Turn emotion into insight.
B1–B3	Be welcome	Accept emotion without suppression.	Transform discomfort into presence.
B4–B6	Benevolence	Respond with empathy and steadiness.	Maintain compassion under pressure.
C1–C3	Control	Regulate body and focus through awareness.	Stabilize the nervous system.
C4–C6	Change	Reprogram emotional habits and thoughts.	Promote neuroplastic adaptation.
D1–D3	Defeat	Deactivate reactive cycles without harm.	Neutralize toxicity.
D4–D6	Dissolve	Release the emotional char-ge and restore calm.	Complete emotional cycles.

14.5 Sample Items by Category

ANTICIPATE: "The Emotional Radar"

1- I notice tension in my body before losing control.

2- I can sense when a conversation is about to turn into conflict.

3- I recognize changes in my breathing or posture when I feel triggered.

Clinical Example:

A high-Anticipation individual might say: "I feel the tightness in my stomach before I react, so now I stop myself". A low-Anticipation person usually realizes it only after the outburst.

ANALYZE: "The Inner Laboratory"

1- When I feel anger or fear, I try to understand what caused it.

2- I can identify repeating emotional patterns in my reactions.

3- I am curious about what my emotions are trying to teach me.

Clinical Example:

An emotionally analytical person might say: "I get angry when I'm ignored because it makes me feel invisible". This cognitive insight reduces reactivity and increases integration.

BE WELCOME: "The Art of Feeling Without Fleeing"

1- I allow myself to feel sadness without trying to push it away.

2- When I'm in pain, I breathe through it instead of distracting myself.

3- I understand that uncomfortable emotions serve a purpose.

Clinical Example:

A patient who says, "Today I allowed myself to cry without judging it", shows the beginning of emotional mastery —acceptance without avoidance.

BENEVOLENCE: "Calm as Strength"

1- I remain calm even when others lose control.

2- I listen fully before reacting or judging.

3- I try to understand others' emotions even when I disagree.

Clinical Example:

A benevolent leader, therapist, or parent creates a **safe physiological environment** —their calm nervous system regulates others through **co-regulation**.

CONTROL: "The Body as a Steering Wheel"

1- I can calm myself using breath or posture.

2- I notice when my body enters tension and can consciously relax.

3- I'm able to pause before responding under stress.

Clinical Example:

An emotionally centered person can stop a panic episode with grounding and breathing, restoring vagal coherence and prefrontal control.

CHANGE: "The Inner Movement"

1- I consciously redirect negative thoughts when they appear.

2- I look for constructive alternatives instead of staying in complaint.

3- I've learned to reinterpret situations that used to paralyze me.

Clinical Example:

A therapeutic turning point occurs when someone shifts from "Why is this happening to me?" to "What can I learn from this?" —activating prefrontal neuroplasticity.

DEFEAT: "Winning without Hurting"

1- I can stop an argument before it escalates.

2- I set clear boundaries without guilt.

3- I don't need to be right to feel at peace.

Clinical Example:

A mature individual doesn't aim to win conversations but to maintain connection.

Defeat in Emotional Aikido means **neutralizing attack without destroying the bond**.

DISSOLVE: "Releasing to Integrate"

1- I know how to close internal or interpersonal conflict without resentment.

2- I can let go of repetitive thoughts that drain me.

3- When something hurts me, I seek to understand it until I can release it.

Clinical Example:
A person with strong dissolving skills can recall a painful event without reliving its physiological distress—their body has released the "sword".

14.6 Scoring and Interpretation

1- Add the three responses for each principle.

2- Divide by 3 to find the **average per domain.**

3- Plot the results in an **eight-point radar chart** (symbolizing the balance of the Aikido circle).

Average	Level	Interpretation
4.5–5.0	Mastery	High coherence, emotional fluency, consistent self-regulation.
3.5–4.4	Functional	Balanced overall, mild reactive tendencies.
2.5–3.4	Developing	Inconsistent awareness, moderate emotional reactivity.
1.0–2.4	Reactive	Difficulty recognizing or managing emotions.

A balanced profile across all eight dimensions reflects **body–mind harmony**. Uneven scores (e.g., high empathy but low control) indicate **imbalances** between openness and regulation.

14.7 Clinical Interpretation Examples

Case A: "The Benevolent Impulsive"

- Anticipate = 2.0
- Analyze = 3.0
- Be Welcome = 4.2
- Benevolence = 4.5
- Control = 2.8
- Change = 3.1
- Defeat = 2.6
- Dissolve = 3.0

Analysis:

High compassion but poor impulse control and anticipation.

Recommendation: train Anticipate and Control (body scans, pre-response breathing, vagal tone exercises).

Case B: "The Rational Controller"

- Anticipate = 4.0
- Analyze = 4.7
- Be Welcome = 2.0
- Benevolence = 2.5
- Control = 4.3
- Change = 3.8
- Defeat = 3.2
- Dissolve = 2.1

Analysis:

Strong cognitive insight but emotional rigidity. The excess of control suppresses affective flow.

Recommendation: enhance Be welcome and Dissolve (acceptance meditation, vulnerability exposure, expressive writing).

14.8 Personal Growth Plan

After scoring, the participant selects for each principle:

- **One daily microhabit.**
- **One weekly practice.**
- **One monthly integration ritual.**

Example:

- **Anticipate:** do a 30-second body scan three times a day.
- **Benevolence:** hold a difficult conversation in a calm tone.
- **Dissolve:** write and tear a symbolic letter of release every Friday.

This transforms the Aikido-IE into a **living training guide**, not just a diagnostic tool.

14.9 Reliability and Validation

The Aikido-IE is currently under **empirical validatio** through multicenter studies. Preliminary pilot results (n = 120) show high internal consistency (Cronbach's α = 0.89) and significant correlations with emotion regulation (*DERS*) and mindfulness (*MAAS*) subscales.

Future research will include **physiological validation** (heart rate variability, galvanic skin response, and fMRI) to integrate subjective and objective emotional regulation metrics.

14.10 Final Remarks

The **Aikido-IE Questionnaire** is not meant to tell you **how emotionally intelligent you are**, but **how harmoniously you flow** with your emotions. It measures the dance between awareness and energy, between control and surrender, between strength and compassion.

Its true purpose is not measurement, but **reflection** to show you the exact point where the art of winning without fighting, the essence of **Emotional Aikido**, begins to unfold within you.

CHAPTER 15.
Neuroemotional Tables

Correlation between neurotransmitters, emotions, and Emotional Aikido techniques

15.1 Neurochemical Foundations of Emotional Flow

Neuro-transmitter	Primary Function	Emotional Aikido Correlation	Deficiency Expression	Techniques That Regulate It
Serotonin	Stability, mood balance	Dissolve	Irritability, insomnia, rigidity	Breath of release, mindful gratitude
Dopamine	Motivation, reward, energy	Change	Apathy, inde-cision	Visualization, small achievements
GABA	Calming inhibition	Control	Anxiety, tension	Slow brea-thing, grounding posture
Oxytocin	Co-nnection, empathy	Benevolence	Isolation, mistrust	Eye contact, compassionate touch

Neuro-transmitter	Primary Function	Emotional Aikido Correlation	Deficiency Expression	Techniques That Regulate It
Norepi-nephrine	Alertness, focus	Anticipate	Fatigue, distraction	Morning body scan, cold exposure
Acetylcho-line	Cognitive clarity	Analyze	Confusion, rumination	Journaling, pattern recognition
Endorphins	Relief, resilience	Defeat	Chronic stress, pain	Movement, laughter, closure rituals
Anan-damide	Emotional integration	Be welcome	Dissociation, emotional numbness	Acceptance meditation, presence in the body

15.2 Neurophysiological Summary

Emotional Aikido works as a **neurochemical harmonizer.** Each discipline stimulates a different system of regulation:

Principle	System Activated	Main Brain Region	Physiological Result
Anticipate	Sympathetic aware-ness	Insula, amygdala	Early detection of stress
Analyze	Cognitive integra-tion	Prefrontal cortex	Emotional insight
Be welcome	Limbic –parasympathetic bridge	Amygdala + vagus nerve	Safe exposure to emotion

Principle	System Activated	Main Brain Region	Physiological Result
Benevolence	Social engagement system	Ventromedial prefrontal cortex	Empathic calm
Control	Autonomic regu- lation	Brainstem + prefrontal cortex	Heart –breath coherence
Change	Neuroplastic circuits	Dorsolateral prefrontal cortex	Rewiring of habits
Defeat	Emotional inhibition	Anterior cingulate cortex	De-escalation
Dissolve	Homeostatic restoration	Hypothalamus + limbic system	Emotional closure

CHAPTER 16.
Clinical and Somatic Protocols

Step by step applications for emotional regulation in clinical practice

16.1 For Anxiety and Panic

1- Postural grounding (feet anchored, exhale twice as long as inhale).

2- Name the body sensations aloud ("Tight chest, fast heart, shallow breath").

3- Introduce rhythmic breathing 4-2-6.

4- After 3 minutes, ask: "What emotion hides beneath the anxiety?"

5- Close with benevolent touch or self-hug to activate oxytocin.

16.2 For Depression or Apathy

1- Movement activation (gentle stretching, slow walking).

2- Dopaminergic stimulation: set one micro-goal and achieve it within an hour.

3- Journaling question: "What am I not expressing?"

4- Gratitude list (3 small things daily).

5- End with 1 minute of open breathing —arms wide, eyes upward.

16.3 For Anger and Irritability

1- Step back physically from the stimulus.

2- Perform the "Breath of Cooling": inhale through nose, exhale slowly through lips.

3- Ask: What am I trying to protect?"

4- Reframe anger as energy for assertive communication.

5- Dissolve with grounding: feel the feet, relax the jaw, lower the shoulders.

16.4 For Trauma and Stress

1- Safety first: create a calm, enclosed space.

2- Practice slow "vagal breathing" (6 breaths per minute).

3- Orient the body: look around the room, notice colors and sounds.

4- Reconnect sensation with words: "I am here now".

5- Close with the Dissolving Breath or minute of silence.

EPILOGUE

"The Path of the Inner Warrior: from Control to Compassion"

The journey of Emotional Aikido ends where it truly begins: in the moment you realize that mastery over emotion is not domination, but **integration**.

Every breath is a chance to return to center. Every emotion is a messenger of transformation. Every act of kindness is a subtle form of victory. The Emotional Aikido practitioner no longer fights their storms; they move through them with grace.

They know that peace is not the absence of struggle, but the ability to remain whole while facing it. And thus, from the dojo of the body to the dojo of life, they carry one final lesson: **to live without resistance is to live in harmony**.

RECOMMENDED READINGS AND SCIENTIFIC REFERENCES

The references constitute the scientific, clinical, and neurophilosophical foundation supporting the models of assessment, emotional regulation, and mind–body integration presented in this work.

Foundational Works

Bradberry, T., & Greaves, J. (2009). Emotional Intelligence 2.0. TalentSmart.

Damasio, A. (1994). Descartes' Error. New York: G. P. Putnam's Sons.

Goleman, D. (1995). Emotional Intelligence. Bantam Books.

Kabat-Zinn, J. (2005). Full Catastrophe Living. Kairós Editorial.

Siegel, D. J. (2012). The Developing Mind. Guilford Press.

Ueshiba, M. (1963). The Art of Peace. Shambhala Publications.

Supplementary Readings

Cozolino, L. (2014). The Neuroscience of Human Relationships. W. W. Norton & Company.

Davidson, R. J., & Begley, S. (2012). The Emotional Life of Your Brain. Hudson Street Press.

Nhat Hanh, T. (2001). Peace Is Every Step. Bantam Books.

Porges, S. W. (2011). The Polyvagal Theory. W. W. Norton & Company.

Van der Kolk, B. (2014). The Body Keeps the Score. Viking Press.

Articles and Scientific Studies

Craig, A. D. (2009). How Do You Feel? Interoception: The Sense of the Physiological Condition of the Body. *Nature Reviews Neuroscience*, *10*(1), 59–70.

Fredrickson, B. L. (2001). The Role of Positive Emotions in Positive Psychology: The Broaden-and-Build Theory of Positive Emotions. *American Psychologist*, *56*(3), 218–226.

Garland, E. L., et al. (2015). Mindfulness-Oriented Recovery Enhancement, Emotion Regulation, and the Neurobiology of Resilience. *Frontiers in Human Neuroscience*, *9*, 386.

Lutz, A., Slagter, H. A., Dunne, J. D., & Davidson, R. J. (2008). Attention Regulation and Monitoring in Meditation. *Trends in Cognitive Sciences*, *12*(4), 163–169.

ANEXXES

ANNEX 1. Medical Aikido Applied to My Emotional Process

Integration worksheet: (*This worksheet is not a test or an assignment. It is a space to support yourself without inner violence*).

Name (optional):______________________________
Date: ____________________________________
Chapter / topic that resonates most with me today:
☐ Anxiety ☐ Depression ☐ Grief ☐ Fear ☐ Guilt ☐ Trauma
☐ Conflicts ☐ Other: ____________________________

1- What am I going through right now?
It doesn't have to be "serious" or clear. Write it as it comes.

____

____

____

2- How does this show up in me?
In my thoughts:
☐ Constant worry.
☐ Rumination.
☐ Guilt.

- ☐ Fear.
- ☐ Confusion.
- ☐ Emptiness.
- ☐ Other:______________________________

In my emotions:

- ☐ Sadness.
- ☐ Anxiety.
- ☐ Anger.
- ☐ Shame.
- ☐ Loneliness.
- ☐ Exhaustion.
- ☐ Numbness.

In my body:

- ☐ Tension.
- ☐ Fatigue.
- ☐ Insomnia.
- ☐ Pressure.
- ☐ Palpitations.
- ☐ Pain.
- ☐ Disconnection.

3- How do I usually respond to this conflict?

- ☐ Avoiding it.
- ☐ Fighting against it.
- ☐ Pushing myself to change quickly.
- ☐ Blaming myself.
- ☐ Trying to control everything.
- ☐ Giving up without care.
- ☐ Observing it from a distance.
- ☐ I don't know yet.

4- Applying Medical Aikido
(Check what feels closest to your experience today).

A- Anticipate · Analyze
When this appears, I usually:
☐ Feel overwhelmed.
☐ Know it's coming.
☐ Go into alert mode.
☐ Recognize it clearly.
☐ I'm not sure yet.

It is usually triggered by:
☐ Thoughts.
☐ Memories.
☐ People.
☐ Situations.
☐ Fatigue/stress.
☐ I don't know.

B- Welcome · Benevolence
Today I can try to:
☐ Stop fighting myself.
☐ Allow the emotion without judging myself.
☐ Remember that feeling is not failing.
☐ Treat myself more gently.
☐ It's still hard for me.

A compassionate phrase I can tell myself today:
☐ "This is difficult, and it's okay that it affects me".
☐ "I don't have to solve everything today".
☐ "I am doing the best I can".
☐ "I am not alone".
☐ Other:

C- Control · Change

Today I can control:

☐ My breathing.
☐ My pace.
☐ What I say or don't say.
☐ Asking for help.
☐ Resting.
☐ Nothing for now, and that's okay.

One small thing I can change today is:

☐ Expecting less from myself.
☐ Listening more to my body.
☐ Not making important decisions.
☐ Setting a boundary.
☐ Giving myself permission to feel.

D- Fall · Dissolve

Today I need to allow myself to:

☐ Not be okay.
☐ Fall a little without guilt.
☐ Cry.
☐ Be in silence.
☐ Not understand everything.
☐ Ask for support.

One inner struggle I can let go of today is:

☐ Having to be strong.
☐ Having to improve quickly.
☐ Having to understand everything.
☐ Comparing myself to others.
☐ Controlling everything.

5- Returning to center
(Coming back to myself, even a little).

I know I'm losing balance when:
☐ My mind won't stop.
☐ My body is tense.
☐ I demand too much of myself.
☐ I isolate.
☐ I react impulsively.

Something that helps me return to center is:
☐ Breathing.
☐ Walking.
☐ Writing.
☐ Talking to someone.
☐ Resting.
☐ Praying/meditating.
☐ I don't know yet.

6-Conscious movement for today
(Choose only one).

Today I practice Medical Aikido by:
☐ Slow breathing for 2-3 minutes.
☐ Moving my body gently.
☐ Writing without correcting myself.
☐ Not demanding results from myself.
☐ Asking for support.
☐ Accepting this moment as it is.

7- Personal closing
Today I don't need to resolve everything. Today I can:

☐ Be with myself.
☐ Rest.
☐ Feel without escaping.
☐ Avoid important decisions.
☐ Trust the process.
☐ Simply exist.

A phrase that helps me today:
☐ "This is a process".
☐ "I don't have to do it perfectly".
☐ "I can go step by step".
☐ "Feeling is not failing".
☐ Other: ______________________________

Final note: Medical Aikido does not seek to eliminate conflict. It helps you move through what hurts without destroying yourself from within.

ANNEX 2 Aikido of Grief. Moving through Loss without Destroying Myself Inside

Integration worksheet (*This worksheet is not about "being okay". It is about accompanying yourself while it hurts*).

Name (optional): ______________________________

Date: ______________________________

The loss I am going through:

(person, relationship, stage of life, health, role, expectation, identity).

____

____

____

1- Which stage of grief do I recognize myself in today?

(This is not a diagnosis. It's a snapshot of the moment).

☐ Denial.

☐ Anger.

☐ Bargaining.

☐ Depression.

☐ Acceptance.

☐ I move between several.

☐ I don't know yet.

This is how this stage feels in me today:

____

____

____

2- How does grief show up in me?

In my thoughts:

☐ "This can't be happening".

☐ Guilt/self-reproach.

☐ "If only I had..."
☐ Repetitive thoughts.
☐ Confusion.
☐ Emptiness.
☐ Other: ______________________________

In my emotions:
☐ Sadness.
☐ Anger.
☐ Anxiety.
☐ Guilt.
☐ Shame.
☐ Loneliness.
☐ Numbness.

In my body:
☐ Fatigue.
☐ Tension.
☐ Insomnia.
☐ Tight chest.
☐ Shortness of breath.
☐ Pain.
☐ Slowness.
☐ Disconnection.

3- How am I responding to this loss?
☐ Avoiding it.
☐ Talking about it all the time.
☐ Getting angry with myself or others.
☐ Trying to understand everything.
☐ Forcing myself to "get over it".
☐ Letting myself fall without care.
☐ Accompanying myself a little.

☐ I don't know yet.

4- Aikido of Grief — how to accompany myself today
(Check what feels closest to your experience).

A- Anticipate · Analyze
When I think about the loss, I usually:
☐ Freeze.
☐ Feel overwhelmed.
☐ Go into alert mode.
☐ Recognize it clearly.
☐ Shift emotions quickly.

What activates my pain the most right now is:
☐ Memories.
☐ Dates/anniversaries.
☐ People or places.
☐ Thoughts.
☐ Fatigue.
☐ I don't know.

C- Be welcome · Benevolence
Today I can try to:
☐ Stop fighting my pain.
☐ Allow myself to feel without judgment.
☐ Remember that grief is not weakness.
☐ Treat myself with more compassion.
☐ It's still hard for me.

A compassionate phrase I can tell myself today:
☐ "This hurts because it mattered".
☐ "I don't have to be okay right now".

☐ "I can go at my own pace".
☐ "Feeling won't break me".
☐ Other: ____________________

D- Control · Change

Today I can control:

☐ My breathing.
☐ My pace.
☐ Who I see/who I talk to.
☐ Asking for help.
☐ Resting.
☐ Nothing today, and that's okay.

One small thing I can change today is:

☐ Expecting less from myself.
☐ Not making important decisions.
☐ Listening more to my body.
☐ Setting a boundary.
☐ Giving myself permission to cry.

E- Fall · Dissolve

Today I need to allow myself to:

☐ Fall a little without guilt.
☐ Not understand anything.
☐ Be sad.
☐ Be in silence.
☐ Remember.
☐ Not function as I used to.

One inner struggle I can let go of today is:

☐ Having to be strong.
☐ Having to "get over it".
☐ Having to be grateful.

☐ Comparing my grief to others.
☐ Controlling my emotions.

5- Returning to center in the middle of grief
(Not going back to who I was before, but coming back to myself).

I know I'm losing my center when:
☐ I disconnect from everything.
☐ I demand too much of myself.
☐ I isolate.
☐ I become emotionally overwhelmed.
☐ I criticize myself for feeling.

Something that helps me return to center is:
☐ Breathing.
☐ Walking.
☐ Writing memories.
☐ Talking to someone safe.
☐ Resting.
☐ Praying/meditating.
☐ I don't know yet.

6- Conscious Aikido of Grief movement (choose one)
Today I practice Aikido of Grief by:
☐ Slow breathing for 2–3 minutes.
☐ Crying without apologizing.
☐ Writing what I miss.
☐ Caring for my body.
☐ Asking for company.
☐ Accepting this moment as it is.

7- Personal closing
Today I don't need to close my grief. Today I can:

- ☐ Accompany myself.
- ☐ Honor what was lost.
- ☐ Rest.
- ☐ Feel without escaping.
- ☐ Stop explaining everything.
- ☐ Trust the process.

A phrase to hold onto today:

- ☐ "Grief is also love".
- ☐ "I'm not breaking, I'm adapting".
- ☐ "I can fall without destroying myself".
- ☐ "This does not define my entire future".
- ☐ Other: ____________________________________

Final note for those going through grief: Grief is not something to defeat or rush. It is something to move through with care. Each time you do not break inside, you are practicing Aikido of Grief.

Annex 3. Emotional Aikido Questionnaire

Based on the 2A + 2B + 2C + 2D system of emotional aikido, this questionnaire was created by Dr. Alexis Gómez González, a graduate of the School of Medical Sciences in Havana and the University of Long Beach, California, with a specialization and master's degree in family medicine and psychiatry.

Administration Instructions:

This questionnaire will help you identify your current level of emotional harmony and your capacity to transform emotional energy into psychophysiological coherence.

Read each statement and mark the option that best describes your habitual behavior (not how you would like to be).

Response Scale

Score	Description
1	Almost never
2	Rarely
3	Sometimes
4	Frequently
5	Almost always

Approximate duration: 8–10 minutes.
Suggested population: adolescents ≥ 16 years and adults.

Answer Sheet

No. – Item – 1 2 3 4 5

Anticipate

1- I notice the early signs of tension in my body before I lose control.

☐ ☐ ☐ ☐ ☐

2- I can recognize when a conversation is about to become conflictive.

☐ ☐ ☐ ☐ ☐

3- I perceive changes in my breathing or posture when something upsets me.

☐ ☐ ☐ ☐ ☐

Analyze

4. When I feel anger or fear, I try to find out what caused it.

☐ ☐ ☐ ☐ ☐

5. I identify patterns that repeat in my reactions.

☐ ☐ ☐ ☐ ☐

6. I am interested in understanding what my emotions are trying to teach me.

☐ ☐ ☐ ☐ ☐

Be welcome

7. I can accept feeling sadness without trying to eliminate it.

☐ ☐ ☐ ☐ ☐

8. When something hurts me, I breathe instead of distracting myself.

☐ ☐ ☐ ☐ ☐

9. I understand that uncomfortable emotions also serve a function.

☐ ☐ ☐ ☐ ☐

Benevolence

10. I respond calmly even when others lose control.

☐ ☐ ☐ ☐ ☐

11. I listen actively before making a judgment.

☐ ☐ ☐ ☐ ☐

12. I try to understand the other person's emotion even when I disagree.

☐ ☐ ☐ ☐ ☐

Control

13. I can calm myself using breathing or by changing my posture.

☐ ☐ ☐ ☐ ☐

14. I notice when my body becomes tense and I consciously relax it.

☐ ☐ ☐ ☐ ☐

15. In moments of stress, I am able to pause before responding.

☐ ☐ ☐ ☐ ☐

Change

16. I try to modify my thoughts when I notice they are negative.

☐ ☐ ☐ ☐ ☐

17. I look for constructive alternatives instead of staying in complaint mode.

☐ ☐ ☐ ☐ ☐

18. I have learned to reinterpret situations that used to paralyze me.

☐ ☐ ☐ ☐ ☐

Defeat

19. I can stop an argument before it escalates.

☐ ☐ ☐ ☐ ☐

20. I know how to set boundaries without feeling guilty.

☐ ☐ ☐ ☐ ☐

21. I do not need to be "right" in order to feel at peace.

☐ ☐ ☐ ☐ ☐

Dissolve

22. I know how to close a conflict without resentment.

☐ ☐ ☐ ☐ ☐

23. I can let go of repetitive thoughts that wear me down.

☐ ☐ ☐ ☐ ☐

24. When something hurts me, I seek to understand it until I can let it go.

☐ ☐ ☐ ☐ ☐

Scoring and Interpretation Sheet

Add the values of each group of three items (per principle).

Divide the total by 3 → average per domain.

Record the results in the table:

Principle	Total Score (3–15)	Average (1–5)
Anticipate		
Analyze		
Be welcome		
Benevolence		
Control		
Change		
Defeat Dissolve		

Annex 4. Aikido-IE Profile Chart (8-domain Radar)

Instructions:

On a circular chart, draw 8 spokes, one for each principle. Mark the average value on each spoke and connect the points:

- A balanced circle indicates emotional harmony.
- An irregular shape shows areas that require strengthening.

General Interpretation:

Average	Level	Description
4.5–5.0	Mastery	High self-regulation, consistent coherence.
3.5–4.4	Functional fluency	Good overall management; mild reactivity.
2.5–3.4	Developing	Emotional inconsistency; practice areas.
1.0–2.4	High reactivity	Difficulty recognizing or regulating emotions.

Personalized Action Plan

After calculating your profile:

1- Identify your two strongest domains → use them as anchors.

2- Select one or two lowest domains → work on them for 4 weeks.

3- Apply the practices recommended in the 12-Week Emotional Aikido Program.

Example:

• If Control and Defeat are low → practice 4-2-6 breathing and compassionate boundaries.

• If Analyze is low → use the "three causes" emotional journaling method.

Emotional maturity is not about feeling less, but about directing the energy of what you feel with wisdom.

Aikido-IE Interpretation with Aikido Belts (Emotional Belts):

Each domain of the Aikido-IE profile offers not only a numerical average, but also a symbolic level inspired by traditional Aikido belts.

This allows you to visualize your progress as a path of discipline, practice, and self-transformation.

Average 1.0– 2.4: White Belt ("Initiation")
Level: High reactivity
Meaning: You are just beginning the path; emotions surprise you or overwhelm you before you can direct them.

Characteristics:

• Low anticipation.
• Difficulty pausing.
• Impulsivity.
• Unclear emotional patterns.

Goal: Develop Anticipate and Control.

Average 2.5–3.4: Blue Belt ("Active Learning")

Level: Developing.

Meaning: There is emotional awareness, but balance is still unstable.

Characteristics:

• Partial mental clarity.
• Intermittent changes.
• Uneven progress.

Goal: Strengthen Analyze, Be welcome, and Change.

Average 3.5–4.4: Brown Belt ("Practical Fluency").
Level: Functional fluency.
Meaning: You manage your emotions well; you recover stability quickly.

Characteristics:

- Good self-regulation.
- Stable empathy.
- Ability to de-escalate conflicts.

Goal: Refine Benevolence, Defeat, and Dissolve.

Average 4.5–5.0: Black Belt ("Inner Mastery")

Level: Mastery.

Meaning: You feel without losing your center; emotional energy is integrated.

Characteristics:

- Excellent bodily anticipation.
- Conscious respiratory control.
- Compassionate communication under pressure.
- Calming influence (co-regulation).

Goal: Maintain harmony and teach others.

Suggested Visual Map for Book/App.

- Anticipate → Brown Belt.
- Benevolence → Black Belt.
- Change → Blue Belt.
- Dissolve → White Belt

The profile becomes a personal emotional dojo.

Official Text to Include:

Emotional Aikido is a path of mastery. Each domain is a belt: you begin in white, advance to blue, flow into brown, and finally integrate black.

It is not about perfection, but about presence.

How the Patient Should Use Emotional Aikido?

Annex 5. Practical Guide and Fallow-up Plan

Emotional Aikido is a daily training system that teaches the patient to recognize, direct, and transform emotional energy by following the eight disciplines of the 2A + 2B + 2C + 2D model:

Anticipate–Analyze–Bewelcome–Benevolence–Control–Change– Defeat–Dissolve

It is not traditional therapy or passive meditation. It is an active, brief, body-oriented method designed to be used in real moments of stress, conflict, or emotional activation.

1. How should the patient practice it?

A. Daily session (5–10 minutes).

A brief routine that includes three essential steps:

Emotional scan (Anticipate)–1 minute.

The patient checks:

- Breathing.
- Posture.
- Muscle tension.
- Current emotional state.

The idea is to notice micro-signals before reacting.

Daily micro-practice (1 technique) – 2 to 4 minutes.

The patient chooses only one technique per day, according to their need:

- 4-2-6 breathing → Control.
- Three Causes Diary → Analyze.
- Somatic acceptance → Be welcome.
- Compassionate phrase → Benevolence.
- 2-minute micro-habit → Change.
- Brief boundary → Defeat.
- Closure practice → Dissolve.

The goal is consistency, not perfection.

Final review (Dissolve) – 1 minute.

The patient evaluates:

- Do I feel calmer?
- What did I learn today?
- Which gate did I work best on?

This reinforces daily integration.

2. How to use it in moments of crisis?

When an intense emotion appears (anger, anxiety, fear, sadness):

5-second pause.

Identify the appropriate gate according to the type of energy:

- Tension → Control.
- Confusion → Analyze.
- Pain → Be welcome.
- Interpersonal conflict → Benevolence or Defeat.

Apply a 1–3 minute technique.

Return to the present.

It is an "emotional first aid" to prevent impulsive reactions.

3. How is progress tracked?

The patient keeps a simple weekly log, which can be done:

- on a sheet of paper.
- in the clinical journal.
- or within the future Aikido-IE app.

Each week they should note:

The gate they practiced the most.

The gate that was hardest.

Real-life moments in which they applied the method.

Changes observed in daily life.

Reactivity level (0–10).

Their emotional belt color (according to averages).

4. Formal evaluation with the Aikido-IE Questionnaire

The patient completes the questionnaire:

- at baseline,
- at 4 weeks,
- at 8 weeks,
- at 12 weeks.

This allows measurement of:

- increased anticipation,
- decreased reactivity,
- improved empathy and communication,
- capacity to close conflicts,
- reduced impulsivity,
- balance among the 8 gates.

The profile is represented with an 8-domain radar graph and an emotional belt.

5. What changes are expected if used correctly?

After 4 weeks:

- Less reactivity,
- Greater body awareness,
- First micro-habits consolidated,

After 8 weeks:

- Improvement in boundaries, communication, and pausing before reacting.
- More consistent self-regulation.

After 12 weeks:

- Integration of the 8 gates.
- Elevated "emotional belt".
- Stable sense of body–mind coherence.
- Better management of interpersonal conflicts.

6. Clinical recommendation

Emotional Aikido works best when combined with:

- psychotherapy (CBT, ACT, DBT),

- physical activity,
- conscious breathing,
- introspective practices.

The physician or therapist should review every 4 weeks:

- which gates improved,
- where blockages remain,
- which techniques work best for that patient,

This way, treatment is personalized.

Summary

Every day you practice one gate.
In every crisis you choose one technique.
Every week you observe your progress.
Every month you evaluate your emotional belt.
That is the path of Emotional Aikido.

Annex 6. Practical Guide to Emotional Aikido for a Work Situation

"A day using Emotional Aikido".

This example shows you how to apply the 2A + 2B + 2C + 2D system in real life, step by step, in everyday situations.

Real situation:

María, 35 years old, feels anxiety and anger because her boss asks her for a report urgently. She already has a heavy workload and feels she will not be able to finish it on time. Her body tenses and she is about to respond impulsively.
Let's see how she applies Emotional Aikido.

1. ANTICIPATE (A)

Internal signal: she notices her chest is tight and her breathing is short. External signal: her boss's tone is dry, fast, pressured.

María thinks: "My body is already warning me. This could end in conflict".

Practice: 10-second body scan.

2. ANALYZE (A)

María asks herself: "What is activating me? Is it really him… or is it my fear of not meeting expectations?" She realizes her mind jumped to: "I won't be able to," "He's going to get angry," "I'm going to fail".

Practice: 30-second mental diary of the three causes:

- Emotional cause: fear of judgment.
- Bodily cause: chest tension.
- Cognitive cause: catastrophic thinking.

3. BE WELCOME (B)

Instead of fighting her anxiety, María thinks: "Okay, I'm anxious. It's okay. I can feel this without running away".

Practice: 20 seconds of gentle acceptance breathing.

Her body begins to lower the alert.

4. BENEVOLENCE (B)

Before answering, María remembers: "My boss is also stressed. It's not personal".

Practice: brief internal empathy phrase: "We both want this to turn out well".

This softens her and avoids confrontation.

5. CONTROL (C)

María does a 4-2-6 breath:

Inhale: 4 seconds.

Hold: 2 seconds.

Exhale: 6 seconds.

Three cycles. Her pulse drops and her body feels more stable.

6. CHANGE (C)

María changes her automatic thought:

Before: "I won't be able to do this" .

Now: "I can divide this into small parts. I'll just start with the first step".

She decides to do a 2-minute micro-habit: organizing the main points of the report.

7. DEFEAT (D)

Here it does not mean "defeat the boss," but to interrupt the toxic cycle.

María sets a compassionate boundary: "I can do it, but I need 40 minutes to reorganize my tasks. I'll send it to you before lunch".

That avoids overload and resentment.

8. DISSOLVE (D)

She ends the interaction and takes a minute to close: "I did the best I could. I released the tension. I'm not holding a grudge".

She takes a long exhale and returns to work without resentment.

What changed with Emotional Aikido?

Before:

- She was about to respond impulsively.
- High anxiety.
- Feeling attacked.
- High risk of interpersonal conflict.

Now:

- She regulated her body.
- She understood her emotion.
- She treated herself kindly.
- She set clear limits.
- She protected her well-being.
- She maintained a stable work relationship.

This is exactly the goal of Emotional Aikido.

Summary for the patient:

When you feel emotionally activated:

1- Notice the signals → Anticipate.

2- Ask yourself what is happening inside you → Analyze.

3- Accept the emotion, do not attack it → Be welcome.

4- Recognize the other person's emotion → Benevolence.

5- Regulate your body with breathing or posture → Control.

6- Change the automatic thought → Change.

7- Break the toxic cycle with healthy limits → Defeat.

8- Close and release the moment → Dissolve.

You cannot always control what you feel, but you can always choose the next movement.

MARÍA (with Aikido-IE scores and belts)

"A day using Emotional Aikido with real scoring".

Real situation:

María, 35 years old, feels anxiety and anger because her boss asks her for an urgent report. She already has a heavy workload and fears she will not be able to complete it. Her body tenses, her breathing changes, and she is about to react impulsively.

Before training Emotional Aikido, María reacted with stress, irritability, and later guilt. Now we will apply the 2A + 2B + 2C + 2D method together with her emotional profile.

1. María's Aikido-IE Score

María completed the questionnaire in Week 0 and obtained:

Anticipate: 3.0 → Blue Belt.

Analyze: 3.8 → Brown Belt.

Be welcome: 2.1 → White Belt.

Benevolence: 3.9 → Brown Belt.

Control: 2.4 → White Belt.

Change: 3.2 → Blue Belt.

Defeat: 2.3 → White Belt.

Dissolve: 2.6 → Blue Belt.

María's global belt: Blue.

(Active Learning Stage: she is no longer at the beginning, but not yet fully fluent).

Her weak areas:

Be welcome, Control, Defeat → White Belt.

Her strengths:

Analyze and Benevolence → Brown Belt.

With this emotional map, let's see how she applies the gates during the conflict.

2. Applying Emotional Aikido in real time

Gate 1: ANTICIPATE (A)

María's belt in this gate: Blue (3.0)

Level: learning, but with partial awareness

Internal signals: tight chest, short breath, warmth in the neck.

External signals: boss's dry, fast, pressured tone.

María thinks: "My body is reacting. This tension is my first signal".

Practice: 10 seconds body scan.

This intervention is successful because she is already at Blue Belt here.

Gate 2: ANALYZE (A)

Belt: Brown (3.8)

Level: very good capacity for self-understanding

María thinks:

"What is activating me so much? Is it him or my fear of not meeting expectations?"

She identifies:

emotion → anxiety.

body → chest tension.

thought → "I'm going to fail".

Practice: mental diary of the three causes.

She manages this gate very well thanks to her Brown Belt.

Gate 3: BE WELCOME (B)

Belt: White (2.1)

Level: initiation; it is hard for her to accept what she feels

Here María usually resists her emotion and wants to "get rid of it".

This time she makes a training effort:

"Okay, I'm anxious. It's okay to feel anxiety. It's not dangerous".

Practice: 20 seconds of gentle breathing.

Because her belt here is White, this part is difficult and not yet automatic. But she manages it.

Gate 4: BENEVOLENCE (B)

Belt: Brown (3.9)

Level: high empathy; strong skill.

María thinks:

"My boss is stressed too. It's not personal".

Practice: Internal empathy phrase: "We both want to solve this".

Thanks to her Brown Belt, this gate comes naturally.

Gate 5: CONTROL (C)

Belt: White (2.4)

Level: high reactivity; low physical regulation.

Before, she would have raised her voice or responded quickly.

Now she applies a brief technique: 4-2-6 breathing for 3 cycles.

Her pulse drops, her mind clears a bit.

The bodily change is key because this is her weakest gate.

Gate 6: CHANGE (C)

Belt: Blue (3.2)

Level: can change thoughts, but not always.

María changes the toxic thought:

Before: "I can't handle this"!

Now: "I'll do it step by step. I'll start with what is essential".

Practice: 2 minutes micro-habit to organize ideas.

Her Blue Belt allows her to shift focus without too much effort.

Gate 7: DEFEAT (D)

Belt: White (2.3)

Level: difficulty setting boundaries.

This is her biggest weakness.

María tends to either give in or explode.

Now she practices a compassionate boundary:

"I can do it, but I need 40 minutes to reorganize my tasks. I'll send it before lunch".

Practice: Brief, kind limit.

It is a major step forward for a White Belt gate.

Gate 8: DISSOLVE (D)

Belt: Blue (2.6)

Level: some capacity to close emotions.

After finishing, she thinks: "I did the best I could. I release the tension".

Practice: Long exhale and emotional closure.

She returns to calm without resentment.

3. Final result using score + belt

Before Emotional Aikido:

- Impulsivity.
- High anxiety.
- Catastrophic thinking.
- Bodily tension.
- Conflict with authority.

After training with her belts:

- She regulated her body (even with a White Belt).
- She accepted her emotion (weak gate).
- She applied empathy (strong gate).
- She changed her thinking (Blue Belt).
- She set healthy limits (big win for a White Belt).
- She closed the conflict without resentment (Blue).

The belt map made it possible to see which gates to use, which would be more difficult, and which could support her.

Emotional Aikido not only tells you WHAT TO DO, but from WHAT LEVEL you are training each skill.

María did not just apply the gates:

- She used her strengths (Brown and Blue Belts).
- She trained her weaknesses (White Belts).
- She regulated a real conflict without losing control.

In the language of the system: She did not react from chaos, but from her emotional map. That is the true progress of Emotional Aikido.

Annex 7. Practical Guide to Emotional Aikido in a Couple Relationship

"A daily conflict that becomes connection".

Situation:

Carlos and Ana have been together for 5 years. Ana comes home upset because Carlos forgot to buy something important at the supermarket.

Carlos is already tired from work and feels "she's attacking me again". They are about to argue. With Emotional Aikido, Carlos changes the course of the conflict. Let's go step by step.

1. ANTICIPATE (A)

Internal signal Carlos notices:

- Tight chest.
- tense jaw.
- Fast thought: "Here we go again… it's about to start".

Before, this tension led him straight to anger.

Now he thinks:

"My body is warning me. If I don't do something, I'm going to react badly".

Practice: 3 conscious breaths.

2. ANALYZE (A)

Carlos asks himself:

"What is really activating me?"

He discovers:

- Fatigue from the day.
- Sense of injustice ("I do a lot").
- Fear of not being enough for her.

Practice: mental diary of the three causes:

- Emotion: irritation.
- Body: tension.
- Thought: "She doesn't value me enough".

3. BE WELCOME (B)

Instead of fighting the emotion, he thinks: "I'm upset and tired. It's okay to feel this. I'm not a robot".

That acceptance reduces about 40% of his impulsivity.

Practice: One long exhale (6 seconds).

4. BENEVOLENCE (B)

Carlos looks at Ana and remembers that she also has her burden.

He thinks:

"It's not against me. She also had a hard day".

This single thought changes his internal tone.

Practice: Active empathy:

"I see you're frustrated, love. Tell me what happened".

Ana softens a bit.

5. CONTROL (C)

Carlos notices his posture is rigid. He relaxes his shoulders and sits down.

Practice: 4-2-6 breathing for 2 cycles.

His body shifts from "fight mode" to "dialogue mode".

6. CHANGE (C)

Instead of thinking, "She's scolding me",
he shifts to: "She wants to feel supported, not attack me".

Practice: Cognitive reframe: "I can listen without defending myself".

7. DEFEAT (D)

Here "defeat" means breaking the automatic toxic argument cycle, not "defeating" the partner.

Carlos calmly says: "I know it bothered you that I didn't buy it. Let me explain what happened without us fighting."

On the other side, Ana drops from 90% reactivity to about 40%.

8. DISSOLVE (D)

After the dialogue and clearing up the misunderstanding, Carlos closes emotionally:

"Thank you for telling me honestly. I don't want this to separate us".

Both feel heard.

Practice: 1 minute of gentle breathing + connection phrase: "We're on the same team".

CONCRETE RESULT

Without Emotional Aikido, this would likely have ended in:

- shouting,
- blame,
- distance,
- accumulated resentment.

With Emotional Aikido:

- there was no shouting.
- both felt validated.
- it was resolved in 3 minutes.
- connection increased.
- Ana ended up saying "thank you".
- Carlos ended in peace, not in guilt.

This is exactly the goal of the method.

SUMMARY

When you have a couple conflict:

1- Feel your body → Anticipate.
2- Observe your emotion → Analyze.
3- Accept it without fighting it → Be welcome.
4- Recognize the other person's emotion → Benevolence.
5- Regulate your body → Control.
6- Change the automatic interpretation → Change.
7- Set a compassionate boundary → Defeat.
8- Close the conflict with connection → Dissolve.

It is not about winning the argument, but about winning the connection.

Annex 8. Example of Scores and Belts in the Couple Relationship

"A daily conflict that becomes connection".

Real situation:

Carlos and Ana have been together for 5 years.

Ana comes home upset because Carlos forgot to buy something important at the supermarket. Carlos is tired from work and feels: "I'm being attacked again". They are seconds away from a major argument. With Emotional Aikido, Carlos transforms the moment.

1. Carlos's Aikido-IE PROFILE (Week 0)

Carlos completes the Aikido-IE Questionnaire and obtains:

Anticipate: 2.8 → Blue Belt.

Analyze: 3.5 → Brown Belt.

Be welcome: 2.2 → White Belt.

Benevolence: 3.7 → Brown Belt.

Control: 2.5 → Blue Belt.

Change: 3.0 → Blue Belt.

Defeat: 2.0 → White Belt.

Dissolve: 2.4 → White Belt.

Global Emotional Belt: Blue (Active Learning).

Strengths:

Analyze (Brown).

Benevolence (Brown).

Intermediate:

Anticipate (Blue).

Control (Blue).

Change (Blue).

Weakest areas:

Be welcome (White).
Defeat (White).
Dissolve (White).

General interpretation:
Carlos is very good at understanding emotions and being empathetic, but struggles to accept his own discomfort, set boundaries without fighting, and close conflicts without holding on to resentment. This is his personal emotional dojo.

2. APPLYING EMOTIONAL AIKIDO DURING THE CONFLICT
They are in the kitchen.
Ana raises her voice.
Carlos feels his body "switch on".
Perfect moment to use the 8 gates of Emotional Aikido.

Gate 1: ANTICIPATE (A).
Blue Belt–2.8
Level: moderate awareness, but not always consistent.
Carlos notices within seconds:
• tight chest,
• tense jaw,
• urge to respond strongly.
He thinks: "My body is warning me. If I don't do something, I'm going to say something I'll regret".

Practice: 3 conscious breaths.
The Blue Belt here helps him stop the automatic reaction.

Gate 2: ANALYZE (A)
Brown Belt: 3.5
Level: strong emotional clarity.

Carlos asks himself:

"What is really activating me?"

He discovers:

- emotion → irritation + fatigue.
- body → tension.
- thought → "Whatever I do is never enough".

Practice: mental diary of de the three causes (10–20 seconds).

The Brown Belt lets him see the root of his reaction without blaming Ana.

Gate 3: BE WELCOME (B)

White Belt: 2.2

Level: beginner; one of his biggest challenges.

Instead of fighting his emotion, he says internally:

"I'm upset and tired. It's okay to feel this".

Practice: One long exhale.

This reduces his reactivity by about 30–40%.

This gate is hard for him because it's a White Belt, but he tries anyway.

Gate 4: BENEVOLENCE (B)

Brown Belt: 3.7

Level: stable empathy when regulated.

Carlos looks at Ana and thinks:

"She is frustrated too. It is not against me".

Practice: Active empathy: "Love, I see you're upset. Tell me what happened".

Ana lowers her defense slightly.

This is a Brown Belt technique: fluid, mature.

Gate 5: CONTROL (C)

Blue Belt: 2.5

Level: moderate ability to regulate the body.

He realizes his posture is rigid.

He adjusts his shoulders and changes his breathing.

Practice: 4-2-6 breathing (2 cycles).

His physiology shifts: from "fight mode" → to "connection mode".

Gate 6: CHANGE (C)

Blue Belt: 3.0

Level: can reframe, although it requires effort.

Old automatic thought: "She's scolding me".

New thought: "She just wants to feel supported".

Practice: Cognitive reframe: "I can listen without defending myself".

This is a solid Blue Belt skill.

Gate 7: DEFEAT (D)

White Belt: 2.0

Level: struggle to stop fights without taking it personally.

This is where he usually explodes.

But now he tries a basic White Belt technique:

Practice: compassionate boundary.

"I know it bothered you that I forgot. Let me explain what happened without us fighting".

He breaks the toxic cycle without attacking.

Gate 8: DISSOLVE (D)

White Belt: 2.4

Level: difficulty closing conflicts.

After clarifying what happened, Carlos does something new:

He does not leave the tension alive.

Practice: Gentle breathing + emotional closing phrase: "I don't want this to distance us. We're on the same team".

The conflict is closed.

3. RESULT OF EMOTIONAL AIKIDO WITH SCORES + BELTS

Before:

- shouting,
- defensiveness,
- blame,
- emotional distance.

With Emotional Aikido:

- no shouting,
- both felt heard,
- mutual empathy,
- healthy boundaries,
- practical solution,
- real connection at the end,
- zero accumulated resentment.

The belts explain why it worked:

His Brown Belts (Analyze, Benevolence) → gave him clarity and empathy.

His Blue Belts (Anticipate, Control, Change) → stopped impulsivity and allowed dialogue.

His White Belts (Be welcome, Defeat, Dissolve) → were exactly where he trained and achieved a new movement.

4. SUMMARY

Carlos did not become a different person.

He simply changed how he moves emotionally.

He identified his belts:

- Brown: where he flows naturally.
- Blue: where he needs consistency.
- White: where he is learning.

In the conflict he:

1- Felt his body.
2- Understood his emotion.
3- Accepted the moment.
4- Empathized with Ana.
5- Regulated his physiology.
6- Changed the interpretation.
7- Set a healthy boundary.
8- Dissolved the conflict.

He did not win the argument. He won the connection.

Annex 9. Clinical Example of how to Calculate the Score

Patient: Laura, 38 years old, teacher, presents with anxiety, irritability, and relationship conflict.

1. Administration of the Aikido-IE Questionnaire

Laura answers the 24 items. Let's assume she gets these scores:

Anticipate (**items 1–3**)

1) **3** 2) **4** 3) **3** → Total = **10**

Average = 10 ÷ 3 = **3.3**

Analyze (**items 4–6**)

4) **4** 5) **4** 6) **5** → Total = **13**

Average = 13 ÷ 3 ≈ **4.3**

Be welcome (items **7–9**)

7) **2** 8) **2** 9) **3** → Total = **7**

Average = 7 ÷ 3 ≈ **2.3**

Benevolence (items **10–12**)

10) **4** 11) **4** 12) **4** → Total = **12**

Average = 12 ÷ 3 = **4.0**

Control (items **13–15**)

13) **2** 14) **3** 15) **2** → Total = 7

Average ≈ **2.3**

Change (items **16–18**)

16) **3** 17) **3** 18) **4** → Total = **10**

Average ≈ **3.3**

Defeat (items 19–21)

19) **2** 20) **2** 21) **3** → Total = 7

Average ≈ **2.3**

Dissolve (items **22–24**)

22) **3** 23) **2** 24) **3** → Total = **8**

Average ≈ **2.7**

2. Belt assignment by domain

Using the interpretation table:

1.0–2.4 → White Belt (Initiation).

2.5–3.4 → Blue Belt (Active Learning).

3.5–4.4 → Brown Belt (Practical Fluency).

4.5–5.0 → Black Belt (Inner Mastery).

It would be:

Anticipate → 3.3 → Blue Belt.

Analyze → 4.3 → Brown Belt.

Be welcome → 2.3 → White Belt.

Benevolence → 4.0 → Brown Belt.

Control → 2.3 → White Belt.

Change → 3.3 → Blue Belt.

Defeat → 2.3 → White Belt.

Dissolve → 2.7 → Blue Belt.

3. Explanation to the patient

As the psychiatrist, you explain it like this:

Laura, this profile is like your "emotional belt map".

It does not say whether you are a good or bad person, but rather what stages you are in for each skill.

For example:

Analyze and Benevolence → Brown Belt.

You already have a good capacity to understand what you feel and to put yourself in others' shoes. You read emotions well and try to be fair.

Anticipate, Change, and Dissolve → Blue Belt.

Here you are in active learning. You already notice that something is moving inside you and sometimes you can change perspective and close conflicts, but not always.

Be welcome, Control, and Defeat → White Belt.

This is where you suffer the most. It is hard for you to allow yourself to feel emotion without fighting it, hard to regulate the body when you are activated, and hard to set boundaries without guilt or stop arguments in time.

This reading lets you tell the patient:

Your problem is not that "you don't have emotional intelligence", but that you are at White Belt in three specific gates. That is trainable.

4. Deciding the "global belt"

You can choose a simple rule:

Option A: average of all domains

Sum of averages:

3.3 + 4.3 + 2.3 + 4.0 + 2.3 + 3.3 + 2.3 + 2.7 = 24.5

Global average = 24.5 ÷ 8 ≈ 3.1 → Global Blue Belt

Option B: clinical judgment

If there are several domains in White and Blue but none in Black, you can say:

"On your overall path you are at Blue Belt: you are no longer starting from zero, but you have not yet consolidated full fluency".

You could summarize it like this:

Global Emotional Belt: Blue (Active Learning).
Strengths: Analyze, Benevolence.
Priority training areas: Be welcome, Control, Defeat.

5. How follow-up works with score and belt

Week 0

The questionnaire is administered.
The belt for each domain and the global belt are determined.
Two gates are chosen to train for 4 weeks (for example: Control and Defeat).

4-week plan for Laura:

Control

Daily 4-2-6 breathing practice 3 times per day.
Body check whenever she feels activated.

Defeat

Compassionate boundary phrases practiced with relationship and work examples.

"Pause before responding" exercises.

Week 4

The Aikido-IE questionnaire is repeated.

Let's assume Control rises from 2.3 to 3.2 (White → Blue). and Defeat rises from 2.3 to 2.8 (White → Blue).

You explain to the patient:

Laura, a month ago you were a White Belt in Control and Defeat.

Today you are already at Blue Belt in both.

That means you still have reactivity, but you are no longer at the level where "emotions run over you"; now you have more capacity for pause and limit.

This generates a very clear and motivating sense of progress: not just "I feel a bit better," but "I have moved up an emotional belt in these two areas".

6. Short explanation example for the patient

Your current profile:

Analyze and Benevolence: Brown Belt.

Anticipate, Change, Dissolve: Blue Belt.

Be welcome, Control, Defeat: White Belt.

In the coming months we are going to work so that your White Belts move up to Blue, and your Blue Belts move closer to Brown.

We are not seeking perfection; we are seeking progress.

You are not your score. Your score is just your training map.

7. How you could include it in the book (brief version for the reader)

Imagine you obtain an average of 2.3 in Control and Defeat: that corresponds to a White Belt. It does not mean you are "bad" as a person, but that you are in the initiation phase of those skills.

Your goal is not to jump straight to Black Belt, but to progress step by step: from White to Blue, from Blue to Brown, from Brown to Black. Every 4 to 8 weeks you can repeat the questionnaire, see your new scores, and check in which domains your emotional belt has changed color.

In this way, Emotional Aikido becomes a measurable path: you do not just feel the change, you can also see it in your profile.

GLOSSARY OF NEUROPHILOSOPHICAL AND EASTERN TERMS

This glossary illustrates how various concepts from Eastern philosophy describe, symbolically and experientially, processes now understood by affective neuroscience, somatic psychology, and modern models of emotional self-regulation.

Term	Meaning	Clinical Translation
Shin-Tai-Ichi	"Unity of mind, body, and spirit"	Somatic–cognitive coherence
Kokyu	"Breath of harmony"	Autonomic balance through rhythmic breathing
Hara	Center of gravity, two fingers below the navel	Core grounding and stability

Term	Meaning	Clinical Translation
Irimi	Entering movement in Aikido	Conscious approach instead of avoidance
Maai	Optimal distance or timing	Emotional boundaries
Kokoro	Heart–mind as a single organ of wisdom	Integration of cognition and emotion
Mushin	"No mind," state of calm awareness	Flow state; absence of over-thinking
Kintsugi	Art of repairing with gold	Transforming wounds into wisdom

These concepts unite Eastern philosophy and modern neuroscience, demonstrating that ancient wisdom anticipated many principles of emotional regulation.

MODERN PSYCHIATRY TOOLS COLLECTION

Each volume in this collection can be read independently, yet together they form a comprehensive clinical system: to evaluate, understand, protect, and regulate the human mind. The books in this series aim to integrate science, clinical practice, and humanity.

The *Modern Psychiatry Tools Collection* was designed to offer clear, practical, and scientifically grounded clinical instruments. Its purpose is to support healthcare professionals in making clinical decisions based on objective evidence.

If this book on *Emotional Aikido* was useful or eye-opening for you, we invite you to explore the other titles, each of these, including this one, has its own English edition.

DNP-21 Model: Neurochemical Profiles and Clinical Algorithms in Psychiatry

This book introduces a brief and structured model for identifying patterns of neurochemical dominance underlying psychiatric symptoms. Rather than merely labeling diagnoses, this instrument helps clinicians understand the patient's functional architecture, enabling more precise, personalized, and safer therapeutic decisions. It is a tool designed for real-world clinical practice, where time is limited and clinical clarity is essential.

PNP-36: Neurochemical Personality Profile

This book expands clinical assessment toward a deeper, dimensional understanding of mental functioning. It presents an extended neurochemical profile that integrates personality, dominant traits, and functional vulnerabilities. Its goal is not to label the patient, but to map their predominant neurobiological style in order to anticipate treatment responses, clinical risks, and more effective therapeutic strategies. It is an advanced tool for clinicians seeking to move beyond isolated symptoms.

EKG Applied to Mental Health

This book addresses one of the most critical and least taught areas in psychiatric practice. It provides a clear and visual guide to understanding the interactions between psychotropic medications and the heart. From QT prolongation to treatment-induced arrhythmias, this text enables clinicians to make safer decisions, anticipate risks, and protect patients. It is an essential tool for practicing responsible and modern psychiatry.

Clinical Laboratory Testing Applied to Psychiatry

This book translates laboratory studies into clinically useful information for assessment, monitoring, and therapeutic adjustment. Hormones, metabolism, inflammation, nutritional deficiencies, and relevant biomarkers are integrated as allies of clinical judgment. The goal is clear: to reduce uncertainty and improve the precision of psychiatric treatment.

Made in the USA
Monee, IL
04 November 2026

67375759R00095